Towards Sustainable Good Health and Well-being

Torstein Hole • Marit Kvangarsnes
Bodil J. Landstad • Elise Kvalsund Bårdsgjerde
Sandra Elizabeth Tippett-Spirtou
Editors

Towards Sustainable Good Health and Well-being

The Role of Health Literacy

Springer

Editors
Torstein Hole
Faculty of Medicine and Health Sciences
Norwegian University of Science
and Technology (NTNU)
Trondheim, Norway

Marit Kvangarsnes
Department of Health Sciences in Ålesund
Norwegian University of Science
and Technology (NTNU)
Ålesund, Norway

Bodil J. Landstad
Department of Health Sciences
Mid Sweden University
Östersund, Sweden

Elise Kvalsund Bårdsgjerde
Department of Health Sciences in Ålesund
Norwegian University of Science
and Techology (NTNU)
Ålesund, Norway

Sandra Elizabeth Tippett-Spirtou
Department of International Business
Norwegian University of Science
and Techology (NTNU)
Ålesund, Norway

ISBN 978-3-031-61809-3 ISBN 978-3-031-61810-9 (eBook)
https://doi.org/10.1007/978-3-031-61810-9

This work was supported by Norwegian University of Science and Technology (981950103).

This Springer imprint is published by the registered company Springer Nature Switzerland AG
The registered company address is: Gewerbestrasse 11, 6330 Cham, Switzerland

Foreword

The 2030 Agenda, also known as the Sustainable Development Goals (SDGs), unanimously adopted in 2015 by all United Nations Member States, provides a comprehensive and collaborative framework for global peace, prosperity, and sustainability.

At its core lies the 17 SDGs, which serve as a clarion call for action by both developed and developing nations. These goals acknowledge the inseparable link between poverty eradication, quality education, reduced inequality, economic growth, environmental preservation, and the improvement of health outcomes.

Central to the agenda is SDG 3, Good Health, and Well-being, which underscores the imperative of accessible healthcare, health promotion, and disease prevention for all individuals.

This book is a call to us all to unite for sustainable health systems. In *Towards Sustainable Good Health and Well-being: the Role of Health Literacy*, we embark on a multifaceted exploration of the intersection between health literacy and the pursuit of sustainable well-being. This book elucidates the pivotal role of health literacy in realizing the ambitions of SDG 3 and advancing broader sustainable development objectives.

To make well-informed and correct decisions about our own health, we all must be able to find, understand, and use health information and services in our respective communities. In other words, we need to make sure that people are health literate. Because only by building health literacy at the micro level, can we assure that Good Health, as defined by Sustainable Development Goal number 3, is achieved on the macro level as well.

Solid systems that prevent the spread of infectious diseases, ensuring universal access to medical care and promoting healthy lifestyles, are fundamental to achieving the global goals. Good national health services for all, global systems for warning of dangers and sharing knowledge, are important. Furthermore, good health and well-being are fundamental prerequisites for people's ability to reach their full potential and to contribute to the development of our societies.

Although our world is currently shifting through difficult times, whether it be climate change or conflict, individuals are seeking ways to live more sustainably. This demand is catalyzing groundbreaking research aimed at revolutionizing health systems. Such innovations promise not only to enhance the sustainability of health services but also to deliver more effective treatments accessible to everyone. This synergy between sustainable living and health-care innovation holds the potential to forge health systems that are not only more environmentally friendly but also more equitable, ensuring that high-quality health care is a universal reality.

Within the context of health literacy, this book highlights the three principles inherent to the SDGs: the Human Rights-Based Approach, Leave No One Behind, and Gender Equality and Women's Empowerment. By embracing these principles, we can address the overall health needs of diverse populations and ensure that no one is excluded on the path toward sustainable good health and well-being.

The transformative ambition and universal applicability of the 2030 Agenda necessitate a steadfast commitment from the United Nations, but also from national governments. This entails upholding international human rights laws, eliminating gender inequalities, and combatting all forms of discrimination. We must prioritize the principle of leaving no one behind, reaching out to those who are most marginalized and disadvantaged, and guaranteeing that everyone can actively participate in and benefit from sustainable development efforts.

In recent decades, historic progress has been made in global health. Nevertheless, the world still has a long way to go to reach future milestones. As the world is currently shaken by unstable and uncertain times, we all have an obligation to fight for a better tomorrow. For a better society for our planet and our children.

This will require major efforts from all of us, throughout all aspects of society, of which good health and well-being is key. We need to do better, be more ambitious, innovative, and learn from each other. This book is an excellent contribution to this mission.

Secretary General, UN Association of Norway — Catharina Bu
Oslo, Norway
March 2024

FN-SAMBANDET
UNITED NATIONS ASSOCIATION OF NORWAY

Acknowledgments

The Editors would like to acknowledge their appreciation for the funding received from the Norwegian University of Science and Technology (NTNU) and Helse Møre og Romsdal Hospital Trust. Without their generous support, this publication would not have been possible.

Introduction

Towards Sustainable Good Health and Well-being: The Role of Health Literacy forms part of Springer's series on Sustainable Development Goals. Springer Nature's inaugural cross-imprint book series addresses and supports the United Nations' (UN) seventeen Sustainable Development Goals (SDGs). This book is divided into three parts that you can either read in continuum, or separately. The chapters follow a deliberate sequence to introduce the reader to the targeted, related, and interconnected topics.

Lack of health literacy continues to be of global concern (WHO 2013; WHO 2021). The European Health Literacy Survey conducted in 2019 provided valuable insights for improving health literacy, preventing disease(s), and promoting better health (WHO 2021). In this book, we address important aspects of health literacy alongside good health and well-being. The book aims to provide new approaches and knowledge for understanding, acting, and assessing health literacy for all.

The book introduces several important concepts required for achieving health literacy and good health and well-being. Patient participation, pedagogical approaches, and patient- and person-centred care will be presented and discussed. Throughout the book we have used the 2020 Centers for Disease Control and Prevention (CDC) definition of health literacy which divides the concept into personal and organisational health literacy.

There are major challenges linked to achieving good health and well-being. The aim of the UN's SDGs is to transform the world. The SDGs are a call to action to end poverty and inequality, protect the planet, and ensure that all people enjoy health, justice, and prosperity. "Leaving no one behind" is an important principle embedded in the SDG goals (United Nations 2015). SDGs comprise a comprehensive framework where the goals are interconnected and integrated: they also need engagement from all perspectives: global, national, and local. The SDGs refer to four distinct areas: human, societal, economic, and environmental, presented as the four pillars of sustainability (United Nations 2015). Primarily the book addresses improving human, as well as social, capital, though the pillars are interconnected. These ideas underpin many of the chapters.

Health literacy is vital for managing health and navigating health services. Personal and organisational health literacy promote sustainability and equity in care and treatment. Literature in this area points out that health literacy is a complex concept because it is both content and context specific (Sørensen 2019). We have addressed different aspects regarding health literacy linked to a range of Sustainable Development Goals (SDGs). The aim is to add new knowledge, tools, and approaches in order to achieve sustainable development for good health and well-being.

This book is divided into three parts as follows: I. Sustainability in Good Health and Well-being, II. Pedagogical Approaches in Building Health Literacy, and III. Experiences of Care and Health Literacy. The three distinct parts present research and systematic work that deals with health literacy and sustainability in good health and well-being. Another common feature is that the chapters focus on both the personal and organisational levels: micro, meso, macro, and exo (Bronfenbrenner 1979). Improving knowledge in these areas is particularly important for strengthening health literacy.

Part I contains three chapters presenting a historical overview (Chap. 1), a comprehensive theoretical model for patient participation (Chap. 2), and an overview of various qualitative designs appropriate for studying health literacy (Chap. 3). This first part aims to provide theoretical approaches and insights into the development of new knowledge about impediments to, and opportunities for, enhancing good health and well-being globally.

The aim of the historical overview in Chap. 1 is to link Sustainable Good Health and Well-being to the Sustainable Development Goals, and to convey a broader overview of how SDGs are interrelated. It also addresses the need to take a multidisciplinary approach to achieve these goals.

A comprehensive theoretical model for patient participation is presented in Chap. 2. The model builds on previous research (Thompson 2007; Thompson et al. 2007) and presents four important factors influencing patient participation: frame factors, interaction, level of involvement, and clinical context. It is intended for use in research and clinical work.

The last chapter of Part I affords the reader with a broad overview of different qualitative research designs that can be used to study health literacy on both personal and organisational levels. Building on this theoretical background, Part II moves on to explore pedagogical approaches for understanding and taking action to improve health literacy.

Part II contains three chapters. Chapter 4 presents a pedagogical model for health professionals to plan, implement, and evaluate pedagogical work to promote health literacy. Chapter 5 provides a potential strategy for supervision in improving good health and well-being. Chapter 6 addresses how to enhance health literacy through sustainable digital healthcare solutions from the perspective of system development and usage. People cannot achieve their optimal or full health potential unless they take charge of factors that determine their health. Pedagogical theories and tools are crucial when attempting to strengthen health literacy and provide more sustainable health services.

Part III contains five chapters that present empirical studies exploring both health professionals' and users' experiences of illness, disabilities, in building health literacy (Chaps. 7, 8, 9 and 10), together with a discussion paper on patient-centred care in a palliative setting (Chap. 11). Health professionals' and users' experiences may provide an opportunity for acquiring additional knowledge about improving patient participation and health literacy during different phases of clinical pathways. Chapter 11 endeavours to explore how health literacy and patient-centred care pathways can improve the quality of care for cancer patients. Patients, users, and health professionals all provide new insights into both the challenges and opportunities which present themselves when trying to improve levels of health literacy.

This book should prove valuable for policymakers, politicians, health managers, health professionals, students and educators within health and social education, patients, users, and family caregivers locally, nationally, and internationally. Our goal is that the book helps to motivate further work to be carried out on improving health literacy and sustainable good health and well-being across theory, practice, and research.

Medical Department, Ålesund Hospital
Møre og Romsdal Hospital Trust
Ålesund, Norway

Faculty of Medicine and Health Sciences
Norwegian University of Science and Technology (NTNU)
Trondheim, Norway

Torstein Hole

Department of Health Sciences in Ålesund
Norwegian University of Science and Technology (NTNU)
Ålesund, Norway

Medical Department, Ålesund Hospital
Møre og Romsdal Hospital Trust
Ålesund, Norway

Marit Kvangarsnes

Department of Health Sciences
Mid Sweden University
Östersund, Sweden

Unit of Research, Education and Development
Östersund Hospital
Östersund, Sweden

Bodil J. Landstad

Department of Health Sciences in Ålesund
Norwegian University of Science
and Technology (NTNU)
Ålesund, Norway

Elise Kvalsund Bårdsgjerde

References

Bronfenbrenner U (1979) The ecology of human development: experiments by nature and design, Harvard University Press, Cambridge, MA

Centers for Disease Control and Prevention (CDC) (2020) What is health literacy. Available: https://www.cdc.gov/healthliteracy/learn/index.html. Accessed 28 Aug 2023

Sørensen K (2019) Defining health literacy: exploring differences and commonalities. In: Okan O et al. (eds.) International handbook of health literacy. Policy Press, The Hague

Thompson A (2007) The meaning of patient involvement and participation in health care consultations: a taxonomy. Soc Sci Med, 64 1297–1310. https://doi.org/10.1016/j.socscimed.2006.11.002

Thompson A et al. (2007) An integrative approach to patient participation in consultations. In: Collins S et al. (eds.) Patient participation in health care consultations qualitative perspectives. Open University Press, Maidenhead

United Nations (2015) Sustainable Development Goals Available: https://sdgs.un.org/goals. Accessed 28 Aug 2023

United Nations (2016) Leaving no one behind: equality and non-discrimination at the heart of sustainable development. Available: https://unsceb.org/sites/default/files/imported_files/CEB%20equality%20framework-A4-web-rev3.pdf. Accessed 21 Feb 2024

United Nations (2022) The Sustainable development goals report 2022. Available: https://unstats.un.org/sdgs/report/2022/The-Sustainable-Development-Goals-Report-2022.pdf. Accessed 28 Aug 2023

WHO (2013) Health literacy The solid facts. Available https://apps.who.int/iris/bitstream/handle/10665/128703/e96854.pdf. Accessed 28 Aug 2023

WHO (2021) Short Summary of the international report on the methodology, results, and recommendations of the European Health Literacy Population Survey 2019–2021 (HLS19) of M-POHL. Available https://m-pohl.net/sites/m-pohl.net/files/inline-files/HLS19%20Short%20Summary.pdf. Accessed 22 Feb 2024

Contents

Contributors

Liv Bakke Outpatient Pain Clinic, Møre and Romsdal Hospital Trust, Ålesund, Norway

Elise Kvalsund Bårdsgjerde Department of Health Sciences in Ålesund, Norwegian University of Science and Technology (NTNU), Ålesund, Norway

Emma Brulin The Department of Occupational Medicine, Institute of Environmental Medicine, Karolinska Institute, Stockholm, Sweden

Augusto Caraceni Università degli studi di Milano, Fondazione IRCCS Istituto Nazionale dei Tumori, Milan, Italy

Berit Misund Dahl Department of Health Sciences, Norwegian University of Science and Technology, Ålesund, Norway
Department of Public Health, University of Stavanger, Stavanger, Norway

Luc Deliens End-of-Life Care Research Group, Vrije Universiteit Brussel and Ghent University, Brussels, Belgium

Marie Fallon Institute of Genetics and Molecular Medicine, University of Edinburgh, Edinburgh, UK

Annik Magerholm Fet Department of International Business, NTNU Ålesund, Ålesund, Norway

Trude Karine Olaug Gjernes Faculty of Social Science, Nord University, Bodø, Norway

Ainhoa Goienetxea Department of Intelligent Production Systems, School of Engineering Science, University of Skövde, Skövde, Sweden

Marianne Hedlund Department of Social Work, Norwegian University of Science and Technology (NTNU), Trondheim, Norway

Erland Hermansen Kysthospitalet in Hagevik, Orthopedic Clinic, Haukeland University Hospital, Bergen, Norway
Department of Clinical Medicine, University of Bergen, Bergen, Norway
Møre og Romsdal Hospital Trust, Ålesund, Norway

Marianne Hjermstad European Palliative Care Research Centre (PRC), Department of Oncology, Oslo University Hospital, and Institute of Clinical Medicine, University of Oslo, Oslo, Norway

Torstein Hole Medical Department, Ålesund Hospital, Møre og Romsdal Hospital Trust, Ålesund, Norway
Faculty of Medicine and Health Sciences, Norwegian University of Science and Technology (NTNU), Trondheim, Norway

Vigdis Schnell Husby Department of Health Sciences, Norwegian University of Science and Technology, Ålesund, Norway
Department of Orthopedic Surgery, Trondheim University Hospital, Trondheim, Norway

Stein Kaasa European Palliative Care Research Centre (PRC), Department of Oncology, Oslo University Hospital, and Institute of Clinical Medicine, University of Oslo, Oslo, Norway

Anniken Karlsen Department of ICT and Natural Sciences, Faculty of Information Technology and Electrical Engineering, Norwegian University of Science and Technology, Ålesund, Norway

Gunhild Hovden Kvangarsnes The National Library of Norway, Oslo, Norway

Marit Kvangarsnes Department of Health Sciences in Ålesund, Norwegian University of Science and Technology (NTNU), Ålesund, Norway
Medical Department, Ålesund Hospital, Møre og Romsdal Hospital Trust, Ålesund, Norway

Bodil J. Landstad Department of Health Sciences, Mid Sweden University, Östersund, Sweden
Unit of Research, Education and Development, Östersund Hospital, Östersund, Sweden

Anne Strand Alfredsen Larsen Department of Health Services Research, Ålesund Hospital, Møre and Romsdal Hospital Trust, Ålesund, Norway

Stig Larsson Department of Clinical Research, Lund University, Malmö, Sweden

Tonje Lundeby European Palliative Care Research Centre (PRC), Department of Oncology, Oslo University Hospital, and Institute of Clinical Medicine, University of Oslo, Oslo, Norway

Synnøve Opsahl Melseth Department of Citizen Services, Ålesund Municipality, Ålesund, Norway

Magne Nylenna Institute of Health and Society, University of Oslo, Oslo, Norway

Anne Lise Sagen-Major Norwegian University of Science and Technology, Ålesund, Norway

Marie Flem Sørbø Department of Public Health and Nursing, Faculty of Medicine and Health Sciences, Norwegian University of Science and Technology, Trondheim, Norway
Competence Centre for Dental and Oral Health, Trondheim, Norway

Amaia Urrizola European Palliative Care Research Centre (PRC), Department of Oncology, Oslo University Hospital, and Institute of Clinical Medicine, University of Oslo, Oslo, Norway

Yan Zhao Faculty of Social Science, Nord University, Bodø, Norway

List of Figures

List of Tables

Part I
Sustainability in Good Health and Well-Being

Chapter 1
Linking Sustainable Good Health and Well-Being to the Sustainable Development Goals: An Historical Perspective

Annik Magerholm Fet

Abstract The aim of this chapter is to provide an overview of the UN Sustainable Development Goals and their relevance for good health and well-being. Sustainable development is defined and then presented within three pillars: social, environmental and economic. The chapter examines these pillars and how they intersect with health.

In 2000, out of the eight Millennium goals launched, six were directed at improving peoples' health whilst the other two focused on environmental sustainability and partnership for development. The 17 SDGs launched in 2015 had 169 targets for 2030: often organised in the so-called *Wedding Cake Model*, which is examined in this chapter. Environmental issues are basic elements in this model, represented by the SDGs 6, 13, 14 and 15. Social issues are tackled through SDGs 1, 2, 3, 4 and 5. All these represent health issues as they relate to goals for "no hunger, education, healthy bodies and gender equality". They are grouped together with SDGs 7, 11 and 16 with focus on access to clean energy, good housing, and strong institutions. The rest of the SDGs (SDGs 8, 9, 10 and 12) are defined as important for the economy (decent work, innovation and infrastructure, equity, responsible consumption and production). Partnership, SDG 17, is the overarching most important SDG, with its main focus on collaboration as a means for achieving a sustainable future. The chapter explores the SDGs for eradicating poverty, combatting inequality and stopping climate change by 2030, all of which impact sustainable good health and well-being.

In conclusion, it addresses the need to take a transdiciplinary approach and forge cross-sectoral and institutional collaboration in order to achieve these SDGs.

Keywords Good health · Well-being · Sustainable Development Goals · Climate change · Transdiciplinary approaches · Sustainability targets · Impact assessment · Environmental impact

A. M. Fet (✉)
Department of International Business, NTNU Ålesund, Ålesund, Norway
e-mail: annik.fet@ntnu.no

T. Hole et al. (eds.), *Towards Sustainable Good Health and Well-being*,
https://doi.org/10.1007/978-3-031-61810-9_1

1.1 Placing the Sustainable Development Goals in Context

The concept of sustainability has developed over time. Over short periods of time, it is difficult to notice specific changes that have taken place, but looking back, we can see that there have been very distinct, and different, eras of change. In the period from the 1850s to the 1960s, pollution and smoke from factory chimneys symbolised industrial growth and prosperity. People flocked from the countryside to the cities to work. Factories were built in ever-increasing numbers across the United Kingdom. In the late 1800s, the impact on the environment magnified. Air quality was affected by smoke, resulting in bodies of water and water sources being polluted. Acidification, fish death and a reduction in biodiversity ensued. As there was a total lack of regulation, emissions quickly spiralled out of control. Populations living in close proximity to provide human resources for industrialisation also resulted in outbreaks of diseases not experienced before, such as the cholera epidemic of 1848 across the United Kingdom. It is difficult to determine how many people died; however, estimates suggest it could have been as high as 50 to 60,000. Poor air quality resulting in "smog" had become commonplace in large cities, such as London, over several hundred years. As industrialization took hold, factories belched out their emissions and people continued to heat their homes with open fires in close quarters, both using cheap coal. The "Great Smog" in 1952 in London lasted 5 days and killed an estimated 12,000 people. This was then followed by the Clean Air Act of 1956, which endeavoured to control domestic sources of air pollution. The Clean Air Act of 1968 was next: it regulated the minimum heights of chimneys, requiring them to be built taller when located nearer to towns. It is clear now that these must have had devastating impacts on peoples' health and well-being, but at the time, it is interesting that factory emissions were not considered significant air polluters.

The focus initially was more on environmental impacts. Environmentalists began to speak out in different ways as time progressed, and the effects on nature were more apparent. For many, Rachel Carson's seminal work, *Silent Spring* (1962), is well known as a catalyst for the environmental movement. It described the use of DDT as a pesticide over large areas in the USA, and how insects and birds were being decimated. Theories about nature's resource limitations were increasingly debated. It was feared that the lack of regulation would lead to resource collapse if the situation was ignored. The period between 1970 and 2000 featured new regulations, standards and practice. Hardin's *Tragedy of the commons* (1968) pointed out the increasing usage of natural resources by industries and the creation of value for industry while the burden of dealing with any environmental issues was left to society and governments. It discussed the importance of joint responsibility for cleaning up damage caused to the environment. *Limits to growth* (Meadows et al. 1972) raised questions about nature's tolerance limit in relation to the extraction of natural resources and pollution. The conclusion was that at least four planets would be needed if we were to continue at the same rate of "progress". The links were clearly made between humans' use of resources, the lack/destruction of them, potential famines and general health and well-being. The inextricable links between human health and ecosystem health are/were there for all to see. The foundation of the environmental movement was built out of concern about the effects of pollution not only on nature, but also on human health.

In 1972, the United Nations Conference on the Human Environment (UNCHE) took place. This conference directed politicians' attention for the very first time to the rising problem of pollution, pesticides and other issues faced on a global scale. There were 113 countries and 400 NGOs present. The Stockholm Declaration on the Human Environment declared that "the natural resources of the earth… must be safeguarded for the benefit of present and future generations" (Principle 3, Environmental Law Guidelines and Principles, The Stockholm Declaration (UNEP 1972).

The United Nations Environmental Program (UNEP) was established at this conference, which signalled the beginning of efforts to protect the global environment. Fifty years of environmental action followed before the celebration in 2022 with examples of action not only globally but also locally (UNCC 2022). In Finland (STUK – Radiation and Nuclear Safety Authority), a division of the Ministry for Social Affairs and Health, for example, had been monitoring the impact of radiation and in particular its use in hospitals since 1958: it was not alone in monitoring nuclear safety.[1] In the USA, the Environmental Protection Agency (EPA[2]) was established in 1970, while in Norway, the Ministry of the Environment was established on 8 May 1972 as the first ministry of its kind in the world, and in 1974, Gro Harlem Brundtland became Minister of the Environment. Denmark quickly followed suit. One of the central tasks was to clean up the pollution problems that the industry had created. It was obvious that water and air were being polluted. Several international conventions were adopted in regard to the environment, for example, the Acid Precipitation Convention in 1979 and the Bern Convention for the Conservation of Biodiversity in 1982. In the early 1980s, the "ozone hole" over Antarctica was discovered and the impact of greenhouse gases and chemical on the atmosphere was assessed, which gave rise to the Montreal Protocol for the Reduction of Ozone-Depleting Gases in 1987. Other examples are the North Sea Declarations for Limiting Emissions in the North Sea in 1988, and the Basel Convention against dumping of toxic waste in the Third World in 1989.

The Brundtland Report *Our common future* (1987) defined the concept of sustainability as follows: "Today's generations must align themselves so that the needs of today's people are met without weakening the basis for future generations to have their needs met". It is recognised as possibly the most quoted definition across the globe. The three pillars, environment, economy and society – also referred to as "people, planet and profit", and part of the definition, were the starting point for discussions at the 1992 Rio Conference. The Rio Declaration on Environment and

[1] Nuclear power, emissions and the use of radiation are not within the scope of this chapter in detail, nor the diverse views on nuclear power in relation to sustainability and sustainable economic development.

[2] https://www.epa.gov

Development (UN 1992) presented 27 principles for a sustainable future, and the meeting resulted in five different documents, amongst which were *the UN Framework Convention on Climate Change, the Convention on Biological Diversity* and in Agenda 21. Agenda 21 comprised a comprehensive plan of action to be taken globally, nationally and locally for the twenty-first century. Agenda 21 and the Commitments to the Rio principles were strongly reaffirmed at the United Nations Conference on Sustainable Development (WSSD) in Johannesburg, South Africa, in 2002, called Rio+10. Hundreds of Heads of State and government and tens of thousands of government representatives and NGOs gathered at this summit.

The United Nations Conference on Sustainable Development (UNCSD) in 2012 (Rio+20) was attended by multinational companies and world leaders. Countries were largely not represented. The ensuing report entitled *The Future We Want* covered broader sustainability topics such as poverty eradication, food security and sustainable agriculture, energy, sustainable transport, sustainable cities, health and population and promoting full and productive employment (UN 2012).

1.2 Sustainable Development Goals and the 2030 Agenda

The current Sustainable Development Goals (SDGs) are officially known as *Transforming Our World: the 2030 Agenda for Sustainable Development.* They include the agreed set of 17 goals and 169 targets from the UN Sustainable Development Summit (2015). The 2030 Agenda for Sustainable Development is "a plan of action for people, planet, prosperity, partnership and peace".

The wedding cake model (Fig. 1.1) shows the three dimensions of sustainability: the biosphere, society and the economy, as being embedded within each other. The environmental aspects in the model are the basic elements, where SDGs 6, 13, 14 and 15 represent access to clean water and sanitation, life below water, life on land and climate action. When considering social issues, SDGs 1, 2, 3, 4 and 5 represent health aspects: no poverty, no hunger, education, healthy bodies and gender equality. These are grouped together with SDGs 7, 11 and 16 which represent access to clean energy, good housing and strong institutions. The remaining SDGs 8, 9, 10 and 12 are defined as important for the economy (decent work, innovation and infrastructure, equity, responsible consumption and production). Number 17, partnership, is at the top, with its focus on collaboration for a sustainable future.

The economic layer sits within the societal layer, which ultimately sits inside the Earth's biosphere. This imparts the irrefutable fact that all activities must be considered within the Earth's system. Interactions between man-made systems – the economic and social layer – and nature are most often represented by flows of materials and resources extracted from nature and emissions, discharges and waste emitted back into natural environmental systems. The impact on nature can be either local, e.g. toxic leakages from landfill, regional, e.g. acidification of earth areas, or global, e.g. emissions of greenhouse gasses (GHGs).

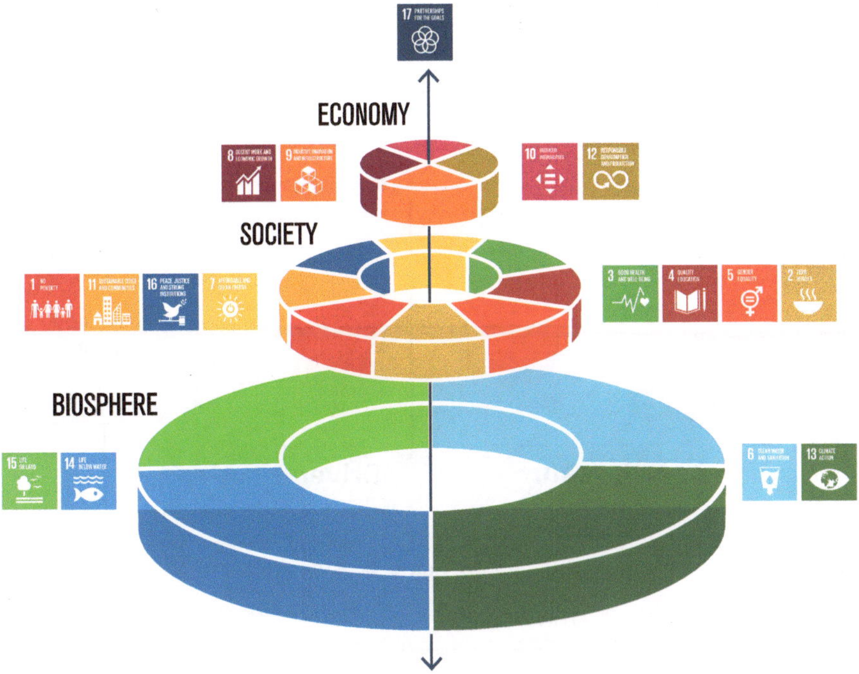

Fig. 1.1 The 17 SDGs presented as the wedding cake model. (Credit: Azote for Stockholm Resilience Centre. Stockholm University CC BY-ND 3.0)

1.3 Impact Assessment Methods

It is important during the transition to sustainable development to establish priorities between different measures to be taken. It is therefore vital to understand impacts on the environment and society, and furthermore, on human health and well-being. There are several methods that can be used to assess such impacts, and in turn, to ascertain which are the most significant. One of the models used on a larger systemic perspective is the DPSIR assessment model. The DPSIR abbreviation is explained in the following text:

D *Driving forces* (population, transport, energy use, industry types, industry structure, land use, landfills, sewage systems)

P *Pressures* (use of resources, emissions, waste generation and noise, radiation, hazards)

S *State* (current state of the quality of air, water and soil quality, ecosystems, biodiversity, vegetation, water organisms, human health)

I *Impacts* (eutrophication, global warming, acidification, poor health conditions in a society)

R *Responses* (prioritising, setting targets, policies, regulations)

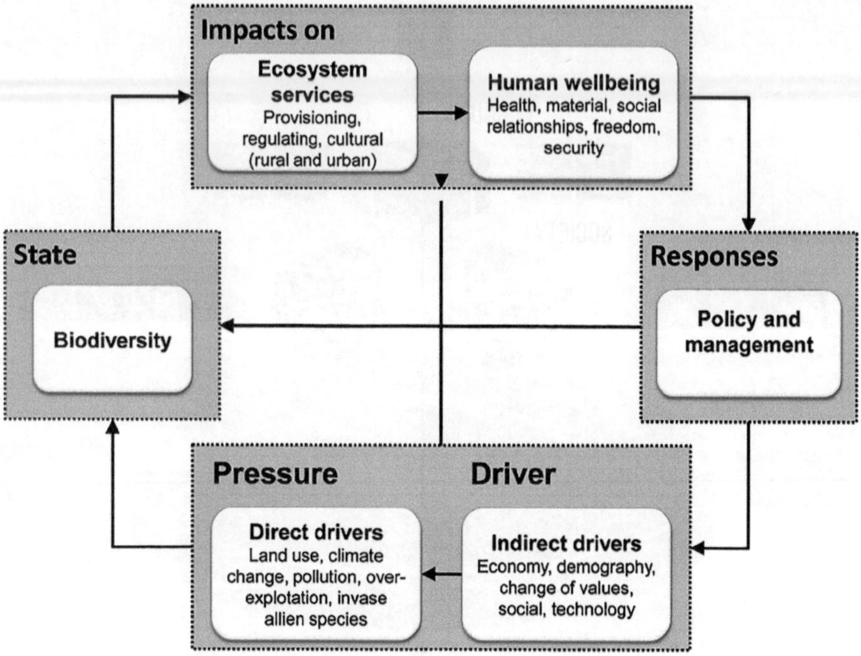

Fig. 1.2 Example of DPSIR with reference to the impact on ecosystem services and human well-being. (Modified from Santos-Martín et al. 2013. Reprinted from Fet, Business Transitions: A Path to Sustainability, Springer 2023)

Figure 1.2 presents an illustration of how the DPSIR framework can be used. Here it is used for a study on drivers that put pressure on biodiversity with an impact on ecosystem services and the resulting consequences for human well-being. The responses here are new policies and regulations to avoid impacts on ecosystem services and human well-being.

There are also various methods which can be used to assess impacts, for example, risk assessments, based on an evaluation of potential accidents and/or emergency situations, or health assessments based upon an evaluation of any changes to health conditions.

In order to evaluate how ecosystem services are affected, a technical process is often used to analyse and assess material flows between nature and man-made systems. The first step is to analyse the material flows in a process, which might be described by the extraction of natural resources or emissions of pollutants to air, soil or water. Generally, further steps involve classification, characterisation and valuation. Classification briefly describes any potential impacts the flows may cause, for example, on global warming, or terrestrial acidification; see left side of Fig. 1.3. The next step, characterization, is a quantitative step in which the relative contributions of the flows are considered for each of the actual impact categories. There are two

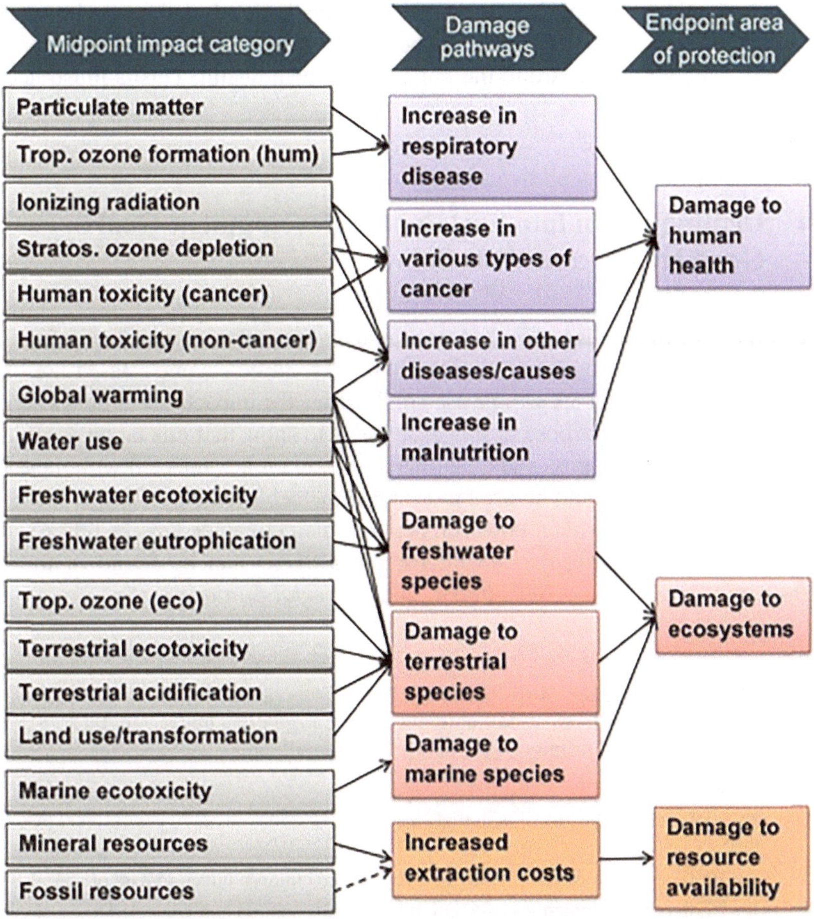

Fig. 1.3 Overview of the impact categories that are covered in the ReCiPe 2016 method and their relation to the areas of protection. The dotted line means there is no constant mid-to-endpoint factor for fossil resources (RIVM 2016) https://doi.org/10.1007/s11367-016-1246-y

mainstream ways to derive characterisation factors, i.e. at midpoint level and at end point level. Whether one decides to consider midpoint or end point consequences is a matter of choice. Emissions of SO_2 or NO_x might be the cause of acid rain which causes terrestrial acidification. This might in turn lead to loss of biodiversity (in this case, in the form of damage to ecosystems). Acidification is defined as a midpoint result, while damage to ecosystem and loss of biodiversity are end point results. The relative importance of different impacts is weighted against each other when the valuation is carried out. Results obtained from the valuation are usually used to prioritise actions, for example, actions by management in an organisation, or recommendations for new regulations.

Evaluation in the impact assessment was originally developed for environmental aspects, however, a similar model can be used for the evaluation of midpoint and endpoint categories in regard to the impact on human health. This is illustrated by Fig. 1.3 (RIVM 2016).

1.4 Drilling Down into Sustainable Development Goal 3: Good Health and Well-Being

The purpose of SDG 3 is to "Ensure healthy lives and promote well-being for all at all ages". It consists of 13 targets (see Table 1.1). Targets named 3a-3d are of an overall character. Target 3.9 will be used to illustrate the impact assessment methods presented above. The purpose of this example is to show that this target is affected by pollution and air quality, and quantitative information connected with measures to reduce pollution, should be used to evaluate the achievement of target 3.9. SDG 3 is used as an example here; however, health is also influenced by the other SDGs, and targets directly linked to health for other SDGs can be found in the UN *Sustainable Development Goals Report 2023: Special Edition.*

Table 1.1 List of targets (https://www.who.int/europe/about-us/our-work/sustainable-development-goals/targets-of-sustainable-development-goal-3) under Goal for SDG 3: Ensure healthy lives and promote well-being for all at all ages

Target	Plan
3.1	By 2030, reduce the global maternal mortality ratio to less than 70 per 100,000 live births.
3.2	By 2030, end preventable deaths of newborns and children under 5 years of age.
3.3	By 2030, end the epidemics of AIDS, tuberculosis, malaria and neglected tropical diseases.
3.4	By 2030, reduce premature mortality by one third.
3.5	Strengthen the prevention and treatment of substance abuse, including narcotic drug and alcohol.
3.6	By 2030, halve the number of global deaths and injuries from road traffic accidents.
3.7	By 2030, ensure universal access to sexual and reproductive healthcare services.
3.8	Achieve universal health coverage.
3.9	**By 2030, substantially reduce the number of deaths and illnesses from hazardous chemicals and air, water and soil pollution and contamination.**
3.a	Strengthen the implementation of the World Health Organization framework convention on tobacco control in all countries.
3.b	Support the research and development of vaccines and access to medicines for all.
3.c	Substantially increase health financing and the recruitment, development, training and retention of the health workforce in developing countries.
3.d	Strengthen the capacity of all countries, in particular developing countries, for early warning, risk reduction and management of national and global health risks.

Modified from *Transforming our world: the 2030 Agenda for Sustainable Development (2023)*

Target 3.9 focuses on the reduction on deaths and illnesses from hazardous chemicals and air, water and soil pollution and contamination. As illustrated in Fig. 1.2, the reduction of ecosystem services can impact human health and well-being. People can also, for example, be exposed to chemicals. This can happen in a working environment where the workforce is exposed to chemicals and other pollutants like noise, dust and vibration. It can also happen later during use of a product in the indoor environment in the home. There is generally no product labelling system that informs the public about exposure from, for example, furniture, clothing or children's toys.

The research project Data Assisted Tools for Sustainable Product Information (DATSUPI) performed by researchers at NTNU in 2005–2009 (Fet and Skjellum 2009) developed a model for how to include data from emissions from materials used during the production of furniture (workplace emissions) and during the use of furniture (indoor emissions). As part of this project, a test program was performed to identify emissions from different materials in furniture. Sixteen tests were performed in a closed test chamber by the accredited laboratory Eurofins in Denmark in 2006–2007, and no people were exposed to chemical or other potential negative health impacts as part of these tests. The results were integrated into a database and used for the purpose of developing health impact categories to be used in the products' label information (Jørgensen 2009, 2013; Fet et al. 2009).

1.4.1 Measuring Damage to Health

There are different models for estimating the potential damage to human health caused by pollution in the air. Harm can be measured in a variety of different ways, depending on the factors involved. Factors can range from variables like types of pollution, types of protection in work environments, status of human health, and which body area is exposed. In a case study on furniture, health-related aspects which were considered the most significant were identified. After this, a set of indicators was suggested and organised systematically. Health effects were measured in relation to the risk posed by exposure to chemicals in the working environment (Skaar and Jørgensen 2013).

Table 1.2 demonstrates the use of indoor environment indices for potential health impacts after using certain products. In the case of furniture, the substances used in their production can impact air quality. Air quality is affected by both volatile and semi-volatile organic compounds, resulting in respiratory health conditions. In conjunction with other chemicals, these impact health and can be a factor in cancer, nephrotoxicity and allergies. The probability of toxicological complications also increases.

The DATSUPI project identified and then classified substances (see Table 1.2). Some materials release unpleasant odours, triggering headaches and general discomfort (Jørgensen 2013).

Table 1.2 Indoor Environment Indices in DATSUPI (Jørgensen 2013)

Index	Classification
Air quality	
Cancer potential	From category 1 (proven carcinogen in humans) to category 3 (concern that the substance is carcinogenic in humans)
Heredity and reproductive harm	From category 1 (proven reduced reproductive capacity, foetal damage or genetic damage in humans) to category 3 (a concern that the substance may cause damage to reproductive capacity, foetus or genetic material)
Allergy potential	Substances with risk phrases R42 or R43 are identified, since they can cause allergies and hypersensitivity in the eyes and respiratory tract or on skin contact
Toxicological potential	

Reprinted with permission from Elsevier from Introduction of a method for presenting health-based impacts of the emission from products, based on emission measurements of materials used in the manufacturing of the products, Environmental Impact Assessment Review, Volume 43, 2013

This section has presented an example of how quantitative information can be gathered from testing, which can also be used to evaluate the achievement of SDG 3, Target 3.9.

1.4.2 Sustainable Development Goal Interactions

The report *A Guide to SDG Interactions: From Science to Implementation* (ICSU 2017) explores interlinkages between the SDGs. It is based on the premise that a science-informed analysis of interactions across SDG domains is essential in supporting more effective decision-making and will thus better facilitate the follow-up and monitoring of progress.

An example of interlinkages between SDGs is shown in a diagram entitled "Interlinkages between Sustainable Development Goals" (ICSU 2017), available at DOI: 10.24948/2017.01. This diagram draws up lines between SDGs 3, 7, 8, 11, 13 and 2. SDG 3 (good health and well-being), target 3.9 (improving health outcomes by improving air quality) is interlinked with SDG 7, since clean energy represents sources with less emissions of pollutants into the air. SDG 2 (zero hunger), target 2.3 (access to sufficient and quality nutrition) is important for good health, and the interaction with SDG 8 (decent work and economic growth) is important for work productivity and health. SDG 11 (sustainable cities and communities) especially targets 11.1 and 11.2 on sustainable urban planning and decent and affordable housing support mental health. SDG 13 (climate action), target 13.2 focuses on the importance between climate change and national policies, strategies and planning, where health concerns are at the centre of decisions made.

In the analyses for the integration of these 5 SDGs, there were 86 target-level interactions, 81 of which were positive and 5 were negative. The analysis concluded that implementing the health dimensions of the SDGs will require the strengthening of national health systems and dedicated laws and regulations to protect people and the natural environment from harmful substances. It will necessitate not only an increased investment in health but also in the infrastructure that supports health and well-being (i.e. sustainable urban design and planning), digital infrastructures, as well as policies that mainstream health concerns from a local (city planning, health and safety in workplaces) to a global scale (preventing and preparing for large epidemics, engaging in multi-stakeholder alliances to tackle antimicrobial resistance, preparing for health impacts as a result of climate change).

The International Science Council[3] which consolidates expertise and advice on matters of global concern to science and society provides a global voice for science. The understanding of possible trade-offs as well as synergistic relations between the different SDGs is crucial for achieving long-lasting sustainable development outcomes. A key objective of the scoring approach described here is to stimulate more science-policy dialogue on the importance of interactions, to provide a starting point for policymakers and other stakeholders to set their priorities and implementation strategies, and to engage the policy community in further knowledge developments in this field (ICSU 2017).

1.5 Transition Instruments

Among other frameworks that support the SDGs is the European Green Deal (EC 2019) with four main goals:

1. EU to become climate neutral by 2050.
2. Protect humans, animals, and plants by cutting pollution.
3. Help companies become world leaders in clean products and technologies.
4. Ensure a just and inclusive transition.

The Green Deal Road Map (EC 2019) made clean energy and zero pollution two of its priorities. Air pollution is the number one environmental health problem in the EU. It causes serious illnesses such as asthma, cardiovascular problems and lung cancer, and vulnerable groups are affected the most. Air pollution also damages the environment and ecosystems through excess nitrogen pollution and acid rain. It is also costly for our economy, as it leads to lost working days and high healthcare costs. To tackle air pollution and achieve the EU's vision of zero pollution for 2050, it has a comprehensive clean air policy based on three pillars: ambient air quality

[3] The International Council for Science (ICSU) and the International Social Science Council (ISSC) merged to the International Science Council (ISC) to provide a global voice for science in 2017.

standards, reducing air pollution emissions, and emission standards for key sources of pollution (EC 2019). **Therefore**, a strategy for the sustainable use of chemicals is part of the European Green Deal plan "A zero pollution Europe".

Similarly, clean, safe and affordable water is essential for peoples' health, and the EU's commitments to the Water Action Plan show its determination to take action for clean water and sanitation for all by 2030. This is also part of the goal of protection of humans, animals and plants by cutting pollution, as is outlined in Goal 2 of that document.

The EU Taxonomy, under the Taxonomy and Transparency Act, emerged from the EU Green Deal initiative as a standardised and comprehensive classification system for sustainable economic activities responsible for up to 80% of EU greenhouse gas emissions (Fet and Sparrevik 2023). These kinds of instruments, which are informative, can raise awareness about the benefits of sustainability through educational programmes. Instruments which are more economic in nature target motivating changes through tax incentives, loan programmes and funding for research programmes or imposing taxes on fossil fuel products or other harmful and hazardous chemicals. The hope is that this will result in not only a cleaner environment, more affordable energy, smarter transport, and new jobs but also an overall better quality of life (Fet and Keitsch 2023).

1.6 Reflections

1.6.1 From Stockholm 1972-Stockholm+50

This chapter started with a review of the background for the SDGs. The UN conference in Stockholm in 1972 was organised as an answer to emerging needs regarding the global state of the environment, as reported from the Stockholm+50 Conference that took place in 2022 (UN 2022). The 1972 conference succeeded in bringing the topic of the environment to the global stage.

The Stockholm Declaration (UNEP 1972) proclaimed:

The protection and improvement of the human environment is a major issue which affects *the well-being of peoples* and economic development throughout the world; it is the urgent desire of the peoples of the whole world and the duty of all Governments.

Since 1972 numerous protocols, conventions and multilateral environmental agreements have been developed. The Rio Declaration, which was a direct outgrowth of the Stockholm Declaration, was adopted in Rio 1992, and Agenda 21 updated the Stockholm Action Plan to address sustainable development issues in the twenty-first century.

The Stockholm+50 conference gave five requirements (UN 2022) for accelerating actions for a Healthy Planet and Prosperity for All. These recommendations are summarised below:

1. Co-working between countries and other stakeholders to address the triple planetary crisis of climate change, biodiversity loss and pollution.
2. Better collaboration and cooperation across environmental efforts within the UN, the private sector and other stakeholders. There is strength in coming together and calling for change.
3. Reinventing an economy for the twenty-first century, e.g. by green or a circular economy; meaning decouple economic development from its destructive footprint.
4. Science, technology and data need to be both accessible and used effectively in addition to strengthening the role of science across the board of enterprises.
5. Raising public awareness about the global nature of environmental problems.

Based on the complexity of these recommendations, it is difficult to design a single straightforward roadmap to deliver the SDGs related to sustainable good health and well-being. However, Stockholm+50 acknowledged the role of the health stakeholder community as more important than ever. They need to be increasingly involved in environmental agendas. Human health and planetary health are seen as synonymous. This interdisciplinary approach was built on the 2015 SDGs which raised environmental issues as part of global economic and health perspectives.

1.6.2 Transition Options to Protect Against Unsustainable Development

The overall vision of the SDGs has been to protect against unsustainable development. Results so far, just over halfway through the 2023 Agenda, demonstrate that protection against degradation of the environment on its own is not enough. Regenerative solutions are required: we must give something better back to nature. Five transition options to facilitate this requirement are suggested by Fet and Keitsch (2023).

The first is *system change*. Society can be viewed as a system with interacting subsystems (e.g. represented by education, health care, industry and government) operating in an environment of common goods where the role of each system element will have an impact on the other. A dynamic understanding of the interaction of systems is based on the insight that much more than incremental changes are needed to depart from the status quo.

The second is *transdisciplinarity*. There is a need for new knowledge where different scientific insights that contribute to both societal and human well-being and scientific progress are integrated. It is important to combine knowledge about nature and the understanding of, for example, air or drinking water quality and its health impact. This chapter presents an example of an impact assessment model as shown in Fig. 1.3. Understanding the mix of consequences on different systems (nature, people, climate, economy, etc.) requires a holistic understanding. Understanding the impact on nature requires competence in the field of natural science, the use of new technologies requires engineering knowledge, the impact on the economy requires social economists, and – last but not least – the impact on human health requires a broad understanding of health issues. The latter involves not only understanding of the effect of different chemicals or other matters on the different parts of the body, but also an understanding the actual long-term impact on human health. This illustrates the vital need for a transdisciplinary approach in dealing with understanding the complexity between SDGs and their actual impact on health because of changes in the environment as seen in Fig. 1.3.

The third option is *net positive leadership*: a way to reinvent the economy for the twenty-first century, for example, by decoupling economic development from its destructive footprint. Target 3.9 under SDG 3 points at the need for action to improve air and water quality for better health conditions, not only reducing the pollution that leads to degradation of air and water quality. Polman and Winston signify sustainability-focused companies as "Net Positive" as it:

> improves well-being for everyone and at all scales – every product, every operation, every region and country, and for every stakeholder, including employees, suppliers, communities, customers, and even future generations and the planet itself. (Polman and Winston 2021).

The fourth recommendation, *digitalization for sustainability*, addresses the need within the UN as well as the private and public sectors for improved collaboration and cooperation on environmental efforts. Digital solutions are seen as a means for getting actions implemented across country borders, e.g. through programmes led by international organisations, but also through artificial intelligence (AI) and data gathering by machine learning and the use of algorithms. Fifty years ago, 113 governments acknowledged the bidirectional relationship between humans and their environment in the Stockholm Declaration. However, in 2022, the global community was perhaps better equipped to practically address this nexus.

The last, *fair and inclusive transitions,* recommends that public awareness should be raised on the global nature of environmental problems. One of the transition instruments in the Green Deal Road Map (EC 2019) is about leaving no one behind. Transition management is seen as essential for directing transformations that support governments in accelerating change towards sustainability and inclusiveness: methodologies for integrating health impacts and well-being with environmental aspects have gained increasing attention. Two global forums with the power of full UN member state participation consider health environment issues on their agendas: the United Nations Environment Assembly (UNEA) and the World Health Assembly (WHA). This bridge is critical, particularly for party-led processes in the UN system. *Governments at large are interested* in this health environment nexus.

The way you manage nature is of course different than that required to manage human health. The core issue is about understanding the intersectionality and managing that (Willetts 2022).

Communities are increasingly encouraging social innovation in order to manage resources for the public good as fairness and inclusiveness are at the very heart of the SDGs.

1.7 Concluding Comments

This chapter has contributed background information to the SDGs and with some reflections around a way to analyse and systematise impacts in general as midpoint and endpoint effects. Damage to human health can be through different damage pathways as illustrated by Fig. 1.3. We cannot ignore the impact of environmental health in our quest to improve human health as described in the goal for 2030: to substantially reduce the number of deaths and illnesses from hazardous chemicals and air, water and soil pollution and contamination.

Through transdisciplinary understanding and new technologies such as AI, we are seeing, and will continue to see, new solutions arising. Interactions between for example SDG 3 and SDG 13 represent opportunities for transdisciplinarity and systems thinking to be used to mitigate climate change and impact on health of future populations. As cross-sectoral and institutional collaboration will become increasingly important if change is to be effective. The following chapters will further illuminate the role of SDGs and their contribution to sustainable good health and well-being.

Appendix

Sustainable Development Goal 3 Targets to Ensure Healthy Lives and Promote Well-Being for All at All Ages

3.1. **Maternal mortality**

By 2030, reduce the global maternal mortality ratio to less than 70 per 100,000 live births.

3.2. **Neonatal and child mortality**

By 2030, end preventable deaths of newborns and children under 5 years of age, with all countries aiming to reduce neonatal mortality to at least as low as 12 per 1000 live births and under-5 mortality to at least as low as 25 per 1000 live births.

3.3. **Infectious diseases**

By 2030, end the epidemics of AIDS, tuberculosis, malaria and neglected tropical diseases and combat hepatitis, waterborne diseases and other communicable diseases.

3.4. **Noncommunicable diseases**

By 2030, reduce by one third premature mortality from noncommunicable diseases through prevention and treatment and promote mental health and well-being.

3.5. **Substance abuse**

Strengthen the prevention and treatment of substance abuse, including narcotic drug abuse and harmful use of alcohol.

3.6. **Road traffic**

By 2020, halve the number of global deaths and injuries from road traffic accidents.

3.7. **Sexual and reproductive health**

By 2030, ensure universal access to sexual and reproductive healthcare services, including family planning, information and education, and the integration of reproductive health into national strategies and programmes.

3.8. **Universal health coverage**

Achieve universal health coverage, including financial risk protection, access to quality essential healthcare services, and access to safe, effective, quality and affordable essential medicines and vaccines for all.

3.9. **Environmental health**

By 2030, substantially reduce the number of deaths and illnesses from hazardous chemicals and air, water and soil pollution and contamination.

Goal 3: Means of implementation for the targets.

3.a. **Tobacco control**

Strengthen the implementation of the WHO Framework Convention on Tobacco Control in all countries, as appropriate.

3.b. **Medicines and vaccines**

Support the research and development of vaccines and medicines for the communicable and noncommunicable diseases that primarily affect developing countries. Provide access to affordable essential medicines and vaccines in accordance with the Doha Declaration on Agreement on Trade-Related Aspects of Intellectual Property Rights (TRIPS) and Public Health, which affirms the right of developing countries to the fullest use of the provisions in the Agreement on Trade-Related Aspects of Intellectual Property Rights (TRIPS) regarding flexibilities to protect public health and, in particular, provide access to medicines for all.

3.c. **Health financing and workforce**

Substantially increase health financing and the recruitment, development, training and retention of the health workforce in developing countries, especially in least developed countries and small island developing States.

3.d. **Emergency preparedness**

Strengthen the capacity of all countries, in particular developing countries, for early warning, risk reduction and management of national and global health risks.

Target 3.8. Universal health coverage

This target can be seen as an overarching one that supports the achievement of the other targets. It is derived from the Millennium Development Goals, the new targets and the means of implementation.

References

Brundtland, G.H., (1987) Our common future: report of the world commission on environment and development. World Commission on Environment and Development

Carson R (2002/1962) [1st. Pub. Houghton Mifflin, 1962]. Silent Spring. Mariner Books

European Commission (EC) (2019) Green Deal Road Map. https://ec.europa.eu/clima/eu-action/european-green-deal_en

Fet AM, Skaar C, Michelsen O (2009) Product category rules and environmental product declarations as tools to promote sustainable products: experiences from a case study of furniture production. Clean Technol Environ 11(2):201–207

Fet AM, Skjellum M (2009) Data assisted tool for sustainability product information (DATSUPI). Main Report, Project no.: 179935/140 NFR, NTNU

Fet AM, Keitsch M (2023) The way forward. In: Fet (ed) Business transition: a path to sustainability – the CapSEM model. Springer, Cham. https://doi.org/10.1007/978-3-031-22245-0_2

Fet AM, Sparrevik M (2023) Reporting schemes. In: Fet (ed) Business transition: a path to sustainability – the CapSEM model. Springer, Cham. https://doi.org/10.1007/978-3-031-22245-0_2

Hardin G (1968) The tragedy of the commons. New Ser 162(3859):1243–1248. (6 pages), American Association for the Advancement of Science

International Council for Science (ICSU) (2017) A guide to SDG interactions: from science to implementation (Griggs DJ, Nilsson M, Stevance A, McCollum D, eds). International Council for Science, Paris. https://doi.org/10.24948/2017.01

Jørgensen R (2009) Testresultater innemiljø, Delrapport i prosjektet «Data assisted tool for sustainability product information (DATSUPI)», in Project no.: 179935/140 NFR, Annik Magerholm Fet, NTNU, Magnar Skjellum, Helland Møbler AS

Jørgensen RB (2013) Introduction of a method for presenting health-based impacts of the emission from products, based on emission measurements of materials used in manufacturing of the products. Environ Impact Assess Rev 43(2013):49–55. https://doi.org/10.1016/j.eiar.2013.05.008

Meadows DH et al (1972) The limits to growth: a report for the Club of Rome's project on the predicament of mankind. Universe Books

Polman P, Winston A (2021) The net positive manifesto, Harvard Business Review Home, the Magazine (September–October 2021). https://hbr.org/2021/09/the-net-positive-manifesto

RIVM, (2016) LCIA: the ReCiPe model, *overview of structure ReCiPe*, a harmonized life cycle impact assessment method at midpoint and endpoint level, report I: characterization, ReCiPe 2016 v1.1, Rijksinstituut voor Volksgezondheid en Milieu/National Institute for Public Health and the Environment, The Netherlands. https://doi.org/10.1007/s11367-016-1246-y

Santos-Martín F et al (2013) Unraveling the relationships between ecosystems and human wellbeing in Spain. PLoS One 8(9):73249. https://doi.org/10.1371/journal.pone.0073249

Skaar, C, Jørgensen, RB (2013) Integrating human health impact from indoor emissions into an LCA: a case study evaluating the significance of the use stage. Int J Life Cycle Assess 18, 636–646 (2013). https://doi.org/10.1007/s11367-012-0506-8
UNEP (1972) Declaration on the human environment (The Stockholm Declaration) (Adopted by the United Nations conference on the human environment, Stockholm, 16 June 1972; see U.N. General Assembly Resolutions 2994/XXVII, 2995/UVII and 2996/XXII of 15 December 1972/(Principle 3, 1972)
UN (1992) The Rio Declaration on Environment and Development
UN (2012) The future we want. United Nations Conference on Sustainable Development
United Nations (2022) The Stockholm +50 Conference, Accessed 20 June 2022. Stockholm+50/ Chasek, P. (Lead author), 2022, United Nations (2022), The Stockholm +50 conference. Accessed DATE, Stockholm+50
UNCC (2022) United Nations Framework Convention on Climate Change: "Fifty years of environmental actions", Jun 3, 2022. https://unfccc.int/blog/fifty-years-of-environmental-action
Willetts L (2022) Stockholm+50: what does it mean for global health. The Lancet Planetary Health 6(5). https://doi.org/10.1016/S2542-5196(22)00100-0

Chapter 2
A Comprehensive Model for Patient Participation

Elise Kvalsund Bårdsgjerde, Marit Kvangarsnes, Bodil J. Landstad, Torstein Hole, and Magne Nylenna

Abstract Patient participation is legislated for internationally and leads to improved patient satisfaction, quality in health services, trust in health professionals, and self-management of disease. Patient participation involves health personnel sharing power, thus empowering the patient. To involve and empower patients is important for achieving several Sustainable Development Goals: Good health and well-being (3) and Reduced equality (10). Patient participation is complex, and the aim of this study is to develop a comprehensive model to understand and improve patient participation in health services and research. Based on 27 qualitative primary studies about patient participation in non-communicable diseases analysed by meta-ethnography, four themes were defined: frame factors, interactions, level of involvement, and clinical context. Including frame factors adds a new dimension to the understanding of patient participation. Frame factors have been underestimated and frame factor theory may be useful to understand and reveal the complexity of patient participation in clinical practice and research.

E. K. Bårdsgjerde (✉)
Department of Health Sciences in Ålesund, Norwegian University of Science and Technology (NTNU), Ålesund, Norway
e-mail: elise.k.bardsgjerde@ntnu.no

M. Kvangarsnes
Department of Health Sciences in Ålesund, Norwegian University of Science and Technology (NTNU), Ålesund, Norway

Medical Department, Ålesund Hospital, Møre og Romsdal Hospital Trust, Ålesund, Norway

B. J. Landstad
Department of Health Sciences, Mid Sweden University, Östersund, Sweden

Unit of Research, Education and Development, Östersund Hospital, Östersund, Sweden

T. Hole
Medical Department, Ålesund Hospital, Møre og Romsdal Hospital Trust, Ålesund, Norway

Faculty of Medicine and Health Sciences, Norwegian University of Science and Technology (NTNU), Trondheim, Norway

M. Nylenna
Institute of Health and Society, University of Oslo, Oslo, Norway

T. Hole et al. (eds.), *Towards Sustainable Good Health and Well-being*,
https://doi.org/10.1007/978-3-031-61810-9_2

Keywords Patient participation · Systematic review · Chronic disease · Health literacy · Sustainable Development Goals · Frame factor theory

2.1 Introduction

Patients have the right to receive information and to participate in decisions regarding their treatment and care (WHO 1994, 2013). Patient participation requires established relationships between patients and health professionals, where they exchange and share information and knowledge, empowering the patients to be able to participate (Cahill 1996; Thompson 2007; Sahlsten et al. 2008). Health literacy is a critical determinant in empowering individuals and enabling their engagement in health and addressing health equity (WHO 2017).

Patient- and person-centred care approaches facilitate patient participation and empowerment (Kitson et al. 2013). Such approaches are important to achieve sustainability in healthcare services (WHO 2017). Improving health literacy in all populations underpins improvements in the Sustainable Development Goals (SDGs), including eradication of poverty and hunger, quality education, and reduced inequalities (WHO 2017; Christie and Ratzan 2019). Health literacy is twofold, and improving health literacy cannot be realised simply through individual actions. It requires health literate–friendly organisations and systems that facilitate improvements in health and well-being for families, communities, and countries (WHO 2017; Christie and Ratzan 2019; Orkan 2019; Sørensen 2019).

Participation means being actively involved in a situation or a matter of importance for those partaking (Oxford English Dictionary 2021). Patient participation and patient involvement are often used synonymously (Cahill 1996; Thompson 2007). Other related terms are patient collaboration, patient partnership, user involvement, user participation, consumer involvement, decision-making, shared decision-making, and empowerment (Arnstein 1969; Brownlea 1987; Cahill 1996; Thompson 2007; Longtin et al. 2010; Vahdat et al. 2014; Castro et al. 2016; Halabi et al. 2020). Patient participation was established as a Mesh term in PubMed in 1978, and there is a great deal of research in the field.

The first framework for citizen participation was developed in 1969 and arranged eight different types of participation in a hierarchy, wherein each type was connected to levels of power. The lowest level is representing non-participation, while the highest level constitutes higher degrees of citizen power and participation in decision-making (Arnstein 1969). Brownlea (1987 p. 605) defined participation as entailing involvement in decision-making processes, in the delivery or evaluation of a service, or simply being consulted on an issue or a matter. Key resources needed for participation to occur are access to appropriate information and knowledge, power, and skills (Brownlea 1987). Although this framework and definition were developed for citizen participation, they have been adapted and applied in developing frameworks for patient participation in healthcare contexts.

Within a healthcare context, patient participation is understood as a mode of social interaction dependent on mutuality between patients and health professionals (Ashworth et al. 1992). Cahill (1996) performed a concept analysis of patient participation within a nursing context. Five attributes were identified in the concept analysis: (1) a relationship between the patient and the nurse must exist; (2) the information, knowledge, and competence gaps between them must be reduced; (3) nurses must release some of their power to the patient; (4) the nurse and the patient must be engaged in intellectual or physical activities; and (5) a positive benefit must occur (Cahill 1996, p. 565). A later concept analysis defined patient participation as an established relationship between patient and nurse based on a surrendering of power and control, sharing of information and knowledge, and reciprocal engagement in an activity (Sahlsten et al. 2008). Cahill (1996) and Sahlsten et al. (2008) have been important contributors to develop the understanding of patient participation in research and nursing practice.

Research on patient participation has developed from describing interactions between patients and health professionals to include the social and structural factors for patient participation (Landstad and Kvangarsnes 2020). Different definitions and theories have been developed to understand patient participation, and extensive research has been conducted to clarify the content of patient participation as a concept (Cahill 1996, 1998; Thompson 2007; Sahlsten et al. 2008; Castro et al. 2016).

A narrative review identified that patient-centred care was dependent on three core elements: patient participation, a relationship between patients and health professionals, and the context of care delivery (Kitson et al. 2013). A concept analysis was conducted aiming to clarify the meaning of the concepts of patient empowerment, patient participation, and patient-centredness. Several similarities were found between the different terms, for example, the balance of power and communication between patients and health professionals (Castro et al. 2016). Halabi et al. (2020) investigated patient participation and the related concepts of patient-centred care, patient empowerment, and patient partnership at the micro-, meso-, and macro levels.

At the micro level, patient participation is characterised by a relationship based on mutual trust, engagement, and open dialogue between patients and health professionals. At the meso- and macro levels, patient participation relied on the structure of the healthcare organisation and system, organisational culture, training, and access to resources (Halabi et al. 2020). Longtin et al. (2010) found that patient participation challenged the paternalistic model in the healthcare system. Patient participation is challenging to achieve in its ideal form, because there will always exist an imbalance in power between patients and health professionals (Angel and Frederiksen 2015). Nurses' and patients' preferences for patient participation may be different; often patients experience participation on a lower or higher level than they prefer (Tobiano et al. 2015).

Patient participation can be promoted or hindered by the characteristics of the healthcare organisation and system (Halabi et al. 2020). Within pedagogy, educational researchers, Urban Dahhlöf and Ulf Lundgren, developed the frame factor theory. The frame factor theory addressed organisational conditions that could either facilitate or hinder learning processes. Examples of frame factors are physical and administrative frames, legislation, and curriculums. Characteristics of frame factors are that they are linked to the system level and may be governed by external conditions (Dahllöf 1967, 1998; Lundgren 1972; Vaage 1998).

Frame factors and the frame factor theory have not hitherto been applied in approaches and models to patient participation (Bårdsgjerde 2022). Andrew Thompson and colleagues have made theoretical contributions by developing a taxonomy and integrative approach to patient participation (Thompson 2007; Thompson et al. 2007). Patient involvement is defined as a complex, multifaceted, and dynamic concept, whereas patient participation is a specific form of involvement based on mutual relationships, dialogue, and shared decision-making when appropriate (Thompson 2007; Thompson et al. 2007).

The taxonomy consists of five levels arranged as follows: "non-involvement", "information-seeking/receptive", "information-giving/dialogue", "shared decision-making", and "autonomous decision-making". The level of involvement is related to the patient's power to influence the situation and varies from non-involvement or exclusion to full autonomy. Patient participation is connected to the level labelled "shared decision-making" and "dialogue" and is dependent on a willingness from both patients and health professionals and a two-way communication characterised by openness and mutual respect (Thompson 2007). The level of involvement is contextual, for example, depending on the type of illness, whether it is acute or chronic, and the severity of the condition. Chronic conditions provide better opportunities for higher levels of patient involvement. The level of involvement is also dependent on patient characteristics and may vary according to circumstances and/or over time for the same person in the same context (Thompson 2007).

The integrative approach shows the multifaceted nature of patient participation and consists of three elements: components, levels, and contexts. The components are (1) patients' contribution to the direction of action, for example, through initiation or response; (2) patients' influence in defining the problem; (3) patients' role in the reasoning process, for example, discussing the issue and its possible solutions; (4) patients' influence in decision-making; and (5) emotional reciprocity between patients and health professionals. The level of involvement often varies within and across these five areas of participation based on the context (Thompson et al. 2007).

Thompson's et al. (2007) integrated approach may be useful for studying patient participation at an individual level. Several recent studies have applied the model as a theoretical framework in studies on participation related to various clinical contexts. The model is valuable to study interactions, but deficient in identifying frame factors' significance on patient participation. Integrating frame factors into the model will provide new knowledge about frame factors that promote and hinder participation. This knowledge can be used to strengthen patient participation in clinical pathways.

2.2 Aim

The aim of this study is to develop a comprehensive model to understand and improve patient participation in health services and research based on empirical research on patient participation and non-communicable diseases (NCDs): cardiovascular disease, cancer, chronic respiratory disease, and kidney disease.

2.3 Method

2.3.1 Design

Meta-ethnography was conducted to synthesise qualitative research (Noblit and Hare 1988). This method involves an interpretive knowledge synthesis where the findings of the included studies are translated into each other and often synthesised in the form of an analogy (Noblit and Hare 1988). The approach is appropriate when the aim is to identify and develop new concepts, theories, and/or models (France et al. 2019).

In conducting this meta-ethnography, we have followed the seven phases developed by Noblit and Hare (1988). Throughout the process, we have applied the Meta-ethnography Reporting Guidance (eMERGe) to inform the design and to ensure complete and transparent reporting (France et al. 2019). Carrying out a meta-ethnography is an iterative process even though the description of the phases may give the impression of a linear process (Noblit and Hare 1988; France et al. 2019).

Phase 1 states a rationale of the study, describes the aim of the study, develops the research (review) question, and explains the appropriateness of conducting a meta-ethnography (Noblit and Hare 1988; France et al. 2019). The rationale of the study has been described in the introduction. To structure the literature search, the following review question was defined: How do patients and health professionals perceive patient participation in various clinical pathways for NCDs?

Phase 2 concerns deciding what is relevant, describing the search strategy and search process, and selecting primary studies. The author group has published articles on patient participation in various clinical pathways. Knowledge of the research field was important when assessing and selecting primary studies. Several of the included studies are authored by the authors of this review.

A librarian assisted in developing the search strategy and structure of the literature search in Medline. The following terms were applied in the initial search: patient participation, consumer participation, patient involvement, patient empowerment, and patient engagement. These terms were combined by using the Boolean "OR". The terms were further combined with the following terms: nurses' attitudes or perceptions, opinions, views, or experiences; physicians' attitudes or perceptions, opinions, views, or experiences; patient perspective or attitudes, perceptions, opinions, views, experiences, or preferences; caregivers' attitudes or perceptions, opinions, views, experiences, or preferences. Combining these terms resulted in 2747 items when the limitations were set to peer-reviewed journals, publication between 2010 and 2023, Danish, English, Norwegian, and Swedish language. These 2747 items were assessed for relevance based on title and abstract. Ninety-five primary research papers were carefully assessed by reading them in full text; 76 articles were excluded, and 19 were included. In addition, we conducted hand searches for articles that did not appear in the database, and another 8 articles were included. The total number of included studies thus became 27. Figure 2.1 shows how the selection of included articles was carried out.

Based on the review question and the aim of the study, we developed the inclusion and exclusion criteria, listed in Table 2.1. These criteria were used to assess the items in the literature search to ensure that included primary studies were able to answer the review question. We assessed the methodological quality of the primary studies by applying the "Consolidated criteria for reporting qualitative research (COREQ): a 32-item checklist for interviews and focus groups (Tong et al. 2007). Studies that did not meet the requirements for quality were excluded. The 95 studies that were read in full text were assessed based on the description of methodology and method. The studies that were included had a clear purpose/research question, and study participants, the context for data collection and data analysis were described. Furthermore, the results section was assessed, and the included studies have rich and detailed descriptions of results underpinned by quotations.

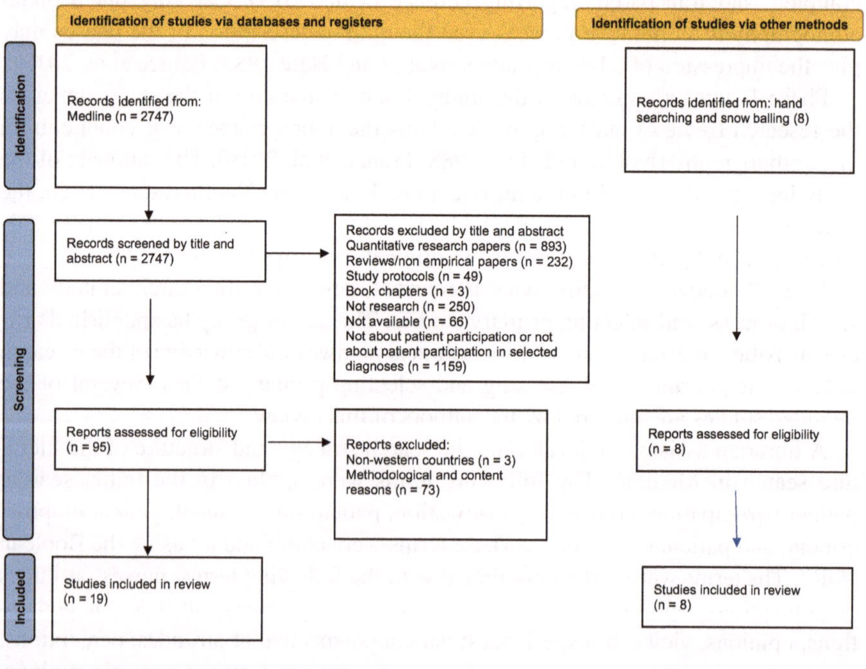

Fig. 2.1 Prisma flow diagram

Table 2.1 Inclusion and exclusion criteria

Inclusion criteria	Exclusion criteria
Empirical research on patient participation	Systematic reviews, non-systematic reviews, concept analyses, and other non-empirical studies
Patient, family caregivers, or health personnel perspective	Other perspectives
Qualitative research	Quantitative research
Non-communicable diseases (NCDs) such as cardiovascular disease, cancer, chronic respiratory disease, and kidney disease	Other diseases
Peer-reviewed and published between 2010 and 2023	Studies published before 2010
Studies conducted in middle- and high-income countries	Studies conducted in low-income countries

2.3.2 Search Outcomes and Quality Assessment

Twenty-seven qualitative studies fulfilled the criteria and were included in this literature review. The included articles are listed in Table 2.2.

2.3.3 Data Analysis

The analysis took place in five steps, phases 3–7, according to Noblit and Hare's (1988) description. In the third phase, the included articles were read to obtain an overview of the themes and metaphors. Then, in the fourth and fifth phases, we decided how the studies were related by comparing patterns and variations in the results.

During this process, the data were coded based on three themes adopted from Thompson et al. (2007) integrative approach to patient participation, including interactions, level of involvement and clinical context. Frame factors were added as a fourth theme. Frame factors are a theoretical approach from the field of pedagogy and were not originally developed within a healthcare context. Frame factors within pedagogy, consisting of physical and administrative frames, legislation, and curriculum design, focus on organisational conditions that could hinder and facilitate learning processes (Dahllöf 1967; Lundgren 1972). Common to these frame factors is that they are linked at the system level and are governed by external conditions that are difficult to control for individuals (Vaage 1998). Similar frame factors are described in literature on patient participation (Bårdsgjerde 2022), and by analysing and synthesising primary research on patient participation we aimed to identify different frame factors at the meso- and macro level and integrate frame factors as a fourth element. The data analysis may therefore be explained as deductive-inductive (Creswell 2014), where we alternated between these four themes and the results of

Table 2.2 Matrix of included studies

First author/year	Country	Title	Data collection	Context	Participants
Aasen et al. (2012a)	Norway	Nurses' perceptions of patient participation in hemodialysis treatment	Individual interviews	Five hospitals in eastern and Western Norway	10 nurses
Aasen et al. (2012c)	Norway	Perceptions of patient participation amongst elderly patients with end-stage renal disease in a dialysis unit	Individual interviews Interview guide with open-ended questions	Five hospitals in Eastern and Western Norway	11 patients
Aasen et al. (2012b)	Norway	The next of kin of older people undergoing haemodialysis: a discursive perspective on perceptions of participation	Individual interviews Interview guide with open-ended questions	Five hospitals in Eastern and Western Norway	7 family caregivers to patients undergoing haemodialysis
Andersen-Hollekim et al. (2019)	Norway	Patient participation in the clinical pathway – Nurses perceptions of adults' involvement in haemodialysis	Focus groups Semi-structured interview guide	Three dialysis units in Central Norway	13 nurses
Andersen-Hollekim et al. (2020)	Norway	Narratives of patient participation in haemodialysis	Individual interviews Interview guide with open-ended questions	Six dialysis units in Central Norway	11 patients
Andersen-Hollekim et al. (2021a)	Norway	Nephrologists' experiences with patient participation when long-term dialysis is required	Individual interviews Semi-structured interview guide	Four dialysis units in Central Norway	10 nephrologists

(continued)

Table 2.2 (continued)

First author/year	Country	Title	Data collection	Context	Participants
Andersen-Hollekim et al. (2021b)	Norway	Shared decision-making in standardized cancer pathways in Norway – Narratives of patient experiences	Individual interviews Semi-structured interview guide	Three University hospitals in Norway	19 patients
Bårdsgjerde et al. (2019)	Norway	Patients' narratives of their patient participation in the myocardial infarction pathway	Individual in-depth interviews	Two cardiac outpatient clinics in Norway	10 patients
Bårdsgjerde et al. (2020)	Norway	Nurses' perceptions of patient participation in the myocardial infarction pathway	Focus groups	Two hospitals in Central Norway	22 nurses
Bårdsgjerde et al. (2022)	Norway	Physicians' perceptions of patient participation in the myocardial infarction pathway	Individual interviews	Two hospitals in Norway	9 physicians
Cohen and Botti (2015)	Australia	Cancer patients' perceptions of the barriers and facilitators to patient participation in symptom management during an episode of admission	Survey with two open-ended questions about patients' perceptions of barriers and facilitators to participate in their symptom management	One hospital in Melbourne, Australia	171 patients

(continued)

Table 2.2 (continued)

First author/year	Country	Title	Data collection	Context	Participants
Höglund et al. (2010)	Sweden	Patient participation during hospitalization for myocardial infarction: Perceptions among patients and personnel	Focus groups Questioning guide	Three hospitals in Stockholm, Sweden	8 patients and 17 health professionals
Ibrahim et al. (2019)	Sweden	"I want to know why and need to be involved in my own care …": a qualitative interview study with liver, bile duct or pancreatic cancer patients about their experiences with involvement in care	Individual interviews Interview guide with open-ended questions	One University hospital in Sweden	20 patients
Jerpseth et al. (2018)	Norway	Older patients with late-stage COPD: Their illness experiences and involvement in decision-making regarding mechanical ventilation and noninvavise ventilation	Individual interviews Semi-structured interview guide using open-ended questions	Three hospitals in Norway	12 patients
Kvangarsnes et al. (2013a)	Norway	Intensive care nurses' perceptions of patient participation in the acute phase of chronic obstructive pulmonary disease exacerbation: An interview study	Focus groups Interview guide with open-ended questions	Two hospitals in Western Norway	17 nurses

(continued)

Table 2.2 (continued)

First author/year	Country	Title	Data collection	Context	Participants
Kvangarsnes et al. (2013b)	Norway	Narratives of breathlessness in chronic obstructive pulmonary disease	In-depth individual interviews Interview guide with open-ended questions	Two intensive care units in Western Norway	10 patients
Landstad et al. (2023)	Norway	Physicians' narratives of communication with patients and their relatives in different phases of the palliative pathway	Individual interviews Interview guide with open-ended questions	Hospitals and primary care settings	13 physicians
Lin et al. (2019)	China	Perceptions of patient participation in symptom management: A qualitative study with cancer patients, doctors, and nurses	Individual interviews Semi-structured interview guide	Two oncological medical units at a hospital in Shanghai, China	41 patients, 5 doctors, and 7 nurses
Netsey-Afedo et al. (2020)	Denmark	No time for reflection: Patient experiences with treatment-related decision-making in advanced prostate cancer	Individual interviews with open-ended questions Participants observations	One urological outpatient clinic at a regional hospital in Denmark	13 patients
Schildmann et al. (2013)	Germany	"One also needs a bit of trust in the doctor…": a qualitative interview study with pancreatic cancer patients about their perceptions and views on information and treatment decision-making	In-depth interviews Semi-structured interview guide	One University hospital in Germany	12 patients

(continued)

Table 2.2 (continued)

First author/year	Country	Title	Data collection	Context	Participants
Svavarsdóttir et al. (2015)	Iceland and Norway	What is a good educator? A qualitative study on the perspective of individuals with coronary heart disease	Individual interviews Semi-structured interview guide	One hospital in Iceland and one hospital in Norway	17 patients
Tarberg et al. (2019)	Norway	Silent voices: Family caregivers' narratives of involvement in palliative care	Individual interviews Interview guide with open-ended questions	Municipalities in mid-Norway	11 family caregivers of deceased cancer patients
Tarberg et al. (2020)	Norway	Nurses' experiences of compassionate care in the palliative pathway	Focus groups Interview guide with open-ended questions	Municipalities in mid-Norway	21 nurses
Tarberg et al. (2022)	Norway	Physicians' perceptions of patient participation and the involvement of family caregivers in the palliative care pathway	Individual interviews Interview guide with open-ended questions	Primary care and hospital	13 physicians
Thaysen et al. (2019)	Denmark	Patient involvement in comprehensive, complex cancer surgery: Perspectives of patients, relatives and health professionals	Individual interviews, focus groups and field observations	Two university hospital surgical departments in Denmark	15 patients, 8 relatives, and 9 health professionals

(continued)

Table 2.2 (continued)

First author/year	Country	Title	Data collection	Context	Participants
Wilson et al. (2017)	Canada	Patient perspectives on engagement in decision-making in early management of non-ST elevation acute coronary syndrome: a qualitative study	Focus groups and individual interviews		20 patients
Årestedt et al. (2019)	Sweden	Patient participation in dialysis care – A qualitative study of patients' and health professionals' perspective	Focus groups	Seven dialysis units at university, county and local hospitals	15 patients, 18 health professionals and 9 managers

the included primary studies. In the sixth and seventh phases, the results from the included studies were synthesised and written in full, illustrated by suitable quotes from the primary studies.

2.4 Results

In the qualitative meta-ethnography synthesis, 27 studies were included. The results are presented in four themes: frame factors, interactions, level of involvement, and clinical context.

2.4.1 *Frame Factors*

Short and fragmented hospital pathways often led to a lack of time and continuity in the patient-health professionals' communication (Bårdsgjerde et al. 2019, 2020, 2022). These frame factors often posed challenges to patient participation:

> First, they are admitted, then they go to the catheterization laboratory and then to the intensive care unit until the evening before they come back to the cardiac ward. And often, the next day, they are discharged (Bårdsgjerde et al. 2020).

Checklists for patient information and involvement across professions and departments were presented as a solution to solve these challenges (Bårdsgjerde et al. 2020, 2022).

Lack of time, continuity, and resources are mentioned as barriers to patient participation in several of the included studies (Höglund et al. 2010; Cohen and Botti 2015; Bårdsgjerde et al. 2019, 2020, 2022; Andersen-Hollekim et al. 2020, 2021a; Landstad et al. 2023). Lack of time, continuity in care, and facilities such as room for private conversations were mentioned as obstacles to patient participation in hospitals (Höglund et al. 2010; Cohen and Botti 2015; Svavarsdóttir et al. 2015; Bårdsgjerde et al. 2022). Frame factors such as time and continuity in care change due to clinical circumstances. In cardiac rehabilitation programmes, health professionals stated that they are provided with better frame factors to facilitate patient participation (Bårdsgjerde et al. 2020, 2022). Illustrated by a quote from one physician:

> After all, patients with MI need cardiac rehabilitation programmes with follow-up over time, because it is all about long-term changes (Bårdsgjerde et al. 2022).

Acute situations often require immediate medical response and decisions in accordance with recommended clinical guidelines (Höglund et al. 2010; Kvangarsnes et al. 2013a; Andersen-Hollekim et al. 2019; Bårdsgjerde et al. 2020, 2022). Health professionals in cardiac care conveyed that standardised recommendations and clear guidelines for acute treatment were often prioritised over patient information and participation in the acute phase (Bårdsgjerde et al. 2020, 2022). Patients' experiences with standardised cancer patient pathways have shown similar findings (Thaysen et al. 2019; Andersen-Hollekim et al. 2021b). From a patient perspective, these pathways seemed to be based on evidence-based knowledge, not requiring patients to be involved in decisions. This is illustrated by the following quote: "It feels like someone has figured out a clever way to do this, and it is thus reasonable to follow this way" (Andersen-Hollekim et al. 2021b). Standardised cancer care pathways led to predictability and safety for the patients.

Tensions and ethical dilemmas arise in the health professional-patient relation in balancing legislated rights, evidence-based healthcare and recognising patients' preferences and values (Aasen et al. 2012c; Kvangarsnes et al. 2013a; Jerpseth et al. 2018; Andersen-Hollekim et al. 2019; Bårdsgjerde et al. 2020; Tarberg et al. 2020; Andersen-Hollekim et al. 2021a; Bårdsgjerde et al. 2022; Tarberg et al. 2022). Health professionals experienced difficult situations during end-of-life care, when elderly and frail patients decline lifesaving treatment such as haemodialysis or percutaneous coronary interventions (PCI) (Aasen et al. 2012a; Bårdsgjerde et al. 2020). This quote illustrates how ethical dilemma may arise between medical knowledge versus patients' preferences: "[…] … It is a treatment offer, but he gets overridden […] We become people of power who dispense our knowledge, without listening to the patient" (Aasen et al. 2012a). Ethical dilemmas often arise in exacerbation of COPD (Kvangarsnes et al. 2013a, b). Nurses have conveyed that they had experiences with using persuasion during acute treatment: "It happens that you have to use a lot of persuasion. Sometimes I've felt that this has been next to using force" (Kvangarsnes et al. 2013a). Within palliative cancer care physicians working in hospitals often experienced that demands for efficiency led to ethical challenges as it hindered them in providing enough time for communication with patients and relatives (Landstad et al. 2023).

Interprofessional collaboration between health professions was emphasised as an important frame factor in several studies. Interprofessional teams, that work together, could contribute to ensuring patient involvement and provide care in line with the patient's needs, wishes, and values (Aasen et al. 2012a; Andersen-Hollekim et al. 2019, 2021a; Bårdsgjerde et al. 2020; Tarberg et al. 2020; Bårdsgjerde et al. 2022; Tarberg et al. 2022).

Patients in need of healthcare services from different departments have highlighted that departments were not coordinated (Andersen-Hollekim et al. 2020). In the palliative care setting, it is important to convey to patients and their family caregivers whether it is the primary or specialist healthcare services that are responsible for the patient's treatment (Tarberg et al. 2022). However, a study from the family caregivers' perspective showed that they often were uncertain about who was responsible for the medical treatment: "I thought it was the physician in the palliative team or in the cancer unit who was in charge and not the family doctor" (Tarberg et al. 2019). The same study revealed that family caregivers often waited too long before they contacted health professionals when the patient's condition altered (Tarberg et al. 2019).

In several studies, health professionals shared reflections about their role as professionals and how the role could influence the level of involvement (Andersen-Hollekim et al. 2019, 2021a). This is illustrated by a quote from a nurse working in a haemodialysis unit:

> I think we have to discuss it. Change the framework. We cannot do things the way we always have … We work quite traditionally. We are the nurses and they are the patients (Andersen-Hollekim et al. 2019).

Interviews with nephrologists revealed that they preferred that the patients were involved in deciding dialysis modality in ample time before initiation. The nephrologists described two different approaches: informed choice and shared decision-making. In the informed choice approach, health professionals provided patients with sufficient information to make a decision themselves, while in the shared decision-making approach, the physicians acted as supervisor, guiding patients towards a choice through dialogue based on the patients' preferences and values (Andersen-Hollekim et al. 2021a). These examples provide an insight into how organisational culture and structure may influence patient involvement. The study conducted by Årestedt et al. (2019) found that the onset of acute dialysis is a point when patient participation is limited, yet patients with a pathway where the illness has manifested gradually may be involved in planning the onset of dialysis.

Health personnel talked about health literate–friendly organisations that strengthened the patient's health literacy and participation in treatment. Studies suggested that some patients were able to administer their own dialysis if they learned how to cannulate the fistula, set up the machine, and run the dialysis session (Årestedt et al.

2019; Andersen-Hollekim et al. 2021a). To enable the patients to participate in their treatment and care might decrease health costs and save staff resources (Andersen-Hollekim et al. 2021a). Another example, illustrating health literate–friendly organisations, is the use of advanced care plans (ACP) in palliative care. Physicians considered ACP as a tool to open and good dialogue including patient and family caregiver's future expectations and their thoughts regarding participation. Patient autonomy was highly emphasised in this process: "It is the patients who own this process" (Tarberg et al. 2022). Patients have expressed that knowledge about how the health system is organised makes it easier for patients to participate (Cohen and Botti 2015).

Several of the included studies highlighted that family caregivers also need information to improve their health literacy and involvement in the patients' treatment and care (Aasen et al. 2012b; Bårdsgjerde et al. 2020, 2022; Tarberg et al. 2020; Tarberg et al. 2022; Landstad et al. 2023). Family caregivers in palliative care experienced the terminal phase as difficult, as they lacked information about what lay ahead and what to expect in this phase of the pathway (Tarberg et al. 2019). Patients have also reported that the involvement of family caregivers facilitated their own participation in care and treatment (Cohen and Botti 2015).

2.4.2 Interactions

Information has been highlighted as an important prerequisite for patient participation (Cohen and Botti 2015; Ibrahim et al. 2019; Lin et al. 2019; Årestedt et al. 2019). Two-way communication is essential, from the health professionals to the patient and vice versa (Lin et al. 2019; Årestedt et al. 2019). Balancing the amount of information has been identified as crucial in several studies (Cohen and Botti 2015; Ibrahim et al. 2019; Årestedt et al. 2019; Netsey-Afedo et al. 2020; Bårdsgjerde et al. 2022). The patients in one study emphasised that the massive flow of information usually left them with no time for reflection (Netsey-Afedo et al. 2020). The terms and language used in information provided by health professionals must be adapted to the patient's level of health literacy (Cohen and Botti 2015; Ibrahim et al. 2019). As illustrated in the following quote: "You have to ask for more information, then you get bombarded with information but not in layman's terms immediately followed by 'any questions?'" (Cohen and Botti 2015).

Several of the included studies provide examples of how patients participate in interactions in various phases of clinical pathways. Patients with renal failure were not involved in deciding whether to start dialysis or in the choice of dialysis options, yet they often were involved during dialysis sessions regarding treatment decisions as how much fluid should be removed and the time spent in dialysis (Årestedt et al. 2019; Andersen-Hollekim et al. 2020).

The studies provide examples that emphasise the importance of interaction through emotional reciprocity in care and treatment. Emotional reciprocity is important in situations where involving patients and family caregivers in medical decisions may not be appropriate (Bårdsgjerde et al. 2019; Bårdsgjerde et al. 2020; Tarberg et al. 2020; Bårdsgjerde et al. 2022; Tarberg et al. 2022). In acute and life-threatening situations, health professionals have to take control and do the best for the patient: "They don't know what's best for them" (Kvangarsnes et al. 2013a).

Patient participation is facilitated through mutual relationships built on trust and respect where the patients are included in the care, listened to, and respected (Cohen and Botti 2015; Svavarsdóttir et al. 2015; Ibrahim et al. 2019; Lin et al. 2019; Årestedt et al. 2019). Patients have expressed that they wish to discuss existential issues with health professionals. Patients being diagnosed with serious illnesses, such as cancer, experienced that the health professionals did not show interest in knowing about their feelings or existential issues (Netsey-Afedo et al. 2020). In palliative care, trust, empathy, and attention were important, and nurses expressed that they emphasised creating a space for dying (Tarberg et al. 2020). Physicians highlighted that in palliative care information meeting the patients' and family caregivers' emotional needs is valuable: "Getting cancer is terrifying and dying is difficult; we all want to live" (Tarberg et al. 2022).

Schildmann et al. (2013) identified that whether patients desired to be involved in treatment decisions at the end of life varied. Health professionals have experienced that it is important to involve patients with COPD in the final stage of treatment decisions. This may lead to a dignified end of life for these patients as illustrated by this dialogue from a focus group with nurses (Kvangarsnes et al. 2013a):

> N7: I have experienced it, but as a wish expressed in a calm and quiet phase [of the disease].
> N8: So, then it was palliative and not curative treatment?
> N7: Yes, and it was all very fine and very dignified, with the family around and a grandchild [performing a] song. And it all turned out to be a fine way of ending life and, in fact, a good memory for the family in the time after.
> N10: Yes, but it is so important that this is clarified in advance.
> N7: Yes.
> N9: Yes, and that it is actually patient participation.

A study revealed that patients in late stages of COPD rarely were involved in decisions regarding their care and treatment. Some of the patients expressed that they wished to discuss the burden versus the benefit of the treatment with health professionals: "Nobody ever talked to me about the disease or the prognosis. Last year I was hospitalized ten times; I tried to talk to the doctors and the nurses, but nobody seemed to want to have such a conversation, so I have given up and stopped asking" (Jerpseth et al. 2018).

2.4.3 Level of Involvement

The studies showed that the level of involvement varied in different phases of the clinical pathways. Trust has been identified as important and may reduce the demand for patient participation in acute and life-threatening situations (Kvangarsnes et al. 2013b; Bårdsgjerde et al. 2019, 2022; Netsey-Afedo et al. 2020).

Health professionals acting with a paternalistic approach in acute situations, which in this case means acting with professionality, being calm, and taking control of the situation, is important for patients to feel safe and trust (Höglund et al. 2010; Kvangarsnes et al. 2013a, b; Bårdsgjerde et al. 2019, 2020, 2022). In addition, to provide patients with short and precise information seems to increase trust in health professionals:

> Even if it was intense situations in the beginning, the people were calm and said what was necessary to say. I think that the way you are met is important in these situations, that they are calm and show that they have control. (Bårdsgjerde et al. 2019)

Studies have shown that trust in health professionals often reduce patients desire to participate in shared decision-making, especially regarding treatment (Kvangarsnes et al. 2013b; Schildmann et al. 2013; Ibrahim et al. 2019; Netsey-Afedo et al. 2020; Andersen-Hollekim et al. 2021b). Taking part in decision-making led to insecurity and the patients did not feel competent to make medical decisions (Ibrahim et al. 2019; Andersen-Hollekim et al. 2021b). The patients wanted to be involved in logistics such as time scheduling and choice of hospital for treatment (Schildmann et al. 2013; Andersen-Hollekim et al. 2021b). Involving patients and their relatives in decisions about medical treatment choices has been expressed as challenging by physicians in palliative cancer care. In such situations, the patients and relatives lacked knowledge and needed experienced physicians to make these decisions and protect them from difficult choices (Landstad et al. 2023).

Health professionals perceived that increased health literacy and involvement have a positive impact on adherence to treatment and lifestyle changes to improve health and well-being (Höglund et al. 2010; Aasen et al. 2012a; Andersen-Hollekim et al. 2019, 2021a; Bårdsgjerde et al. 2020, 2022). Self-management requires patients with sufficient health literacy to understand why it is important to adhere to lifestyle changes, including specific diets, fluid restrictions, and physical activity, and to administer medications as prescribed (Andersen-Hollekim et al. 2021a; Bårdsgjerde et al. 2022). Elderly patients expressed that they often negotiated between maintaining a good quality of life today and having a "long life", considering how strictly they adhered to fluid and dietary restrictions (Aasen et al. 2012c).

2.4.4 Clinical Context

The studies showed that the level of involvement depended on the context. There is less need for participation in acute situations versus stable phases of disease. In acute situations, patients need short and clear information, provided through one-way communication from health professionals to patients (Höglund et al. 2010; Kvangarsnes et al. 2013a; Wilson et al. 2017; Bårdsgjerde et al. 2019, 2020, 2022).

During long-term treatment, patients desire to be involved in their care and treatment (Höglund et al. 2010; Schildmann et al. 2013; Wilson et al. 2017). Physicians conveyed that the patients wanted to be involved in decisions about the prescription of medications (Bårdsgjerde et al. 2022). Patient participation in decisions requires patients who are health literate: "If the patients are supposed to take part in decisions, it requires a great deal of information and that the patients really understand the information they have received" (Bårdsgjerde et al. 2020). Low levels of health literacy could hinder shared decision-making and may lead to health professionals making decisions on behalf of patients (Andersen-Hollekim et al. 2019; Bårdsgjerde et al. 2020).

Attending cardiac rehabilitation programmes seems to increase the patient's health literacy, which leads to patients participating at a higher level for improving their health and achieving control over risk factors. As stated by one patient: "I have received most information through this course, they have told us about the heart's physiology and its function, diets and exercise" (Bårdsgjerde et al. 2019). Yet, sufficient health literacy is not equal to increased involvement. Patients with renal failure conveyed that they were well informed before the initiation of dialysis, and yet they were still not involved in decisions regarding dialysis options (Andersen-Hollekim et al. 2020).

The importance of involving family caregivers as a resource for patients was pointed out in studies from the perspectives of health professionals (Kvangarsnes et al. 2013a; Cohen and Botti 2015; Andersen-Hollekim et al. 2019; Bårdsgjerde et al. 2020, 2022; Tarberg et al. 2020; Tarberg et al. 2022; Landstad et al. 2023). Especially, in palliative care, involving family caregivers was seen as a prerequisite when death at home was planned (Tarberg et al. 2022). Studies from the family caregivers' perspective, however, showed that they often felt left out in the decision to plan for death at home: "He decided. He let us know early on that he wanted to stay home". In some cases, family caregivers felt that they had too much responsibility and expressed concern about how best to bear the burden (Tarberg et al. 2019).

Studies have revealed that health professionals and family caregivers experience challenges in the involvement of family caregivers (Aasen et al. 2012a, b; Andersen-Hollekim et al. 2019; Tarberg et al. 2019, 2020, 2022; Bårdsgjerde et al. 2020, 2022). Health professionals have reported that family caregivers are little involved in dialysis treatment (Aasen et al. 2012a; Andersen-Hollekim et al. 2019). Family caregivers expressed that they felt forgotten and not involved when someone in their family was undergoing dialysis (Aasen et al. 2012b). In palliative care, family caregivers are often in need of information and dialogue with health professionals without the patient present. They experienced that it was difficult to ask for this information: "That would mean you want to talk about something that you can't address with the patient present" (Tarberg et al. 2019).

2.5 Discussion

Based on the synthesis of previous research and pedagogical theory, we have developed a comprehensive model for patient participation (Fig. 2.2). In this model, we present the four themes in Sect. 2.4 using sub-themes relevant to understanding

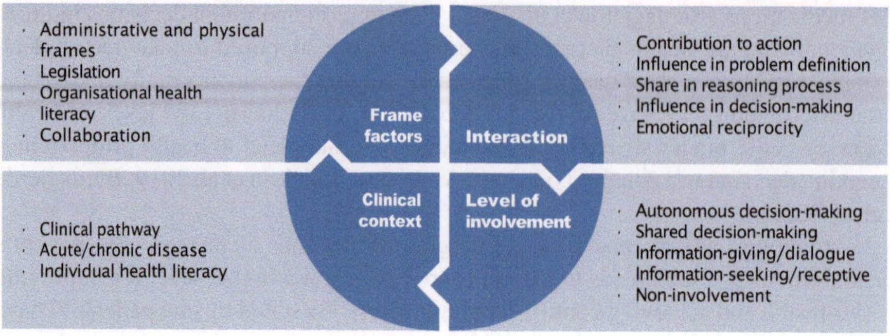

Fig. 2.2 Modified from "Perceptions of Patient Participation in the Myocardial Infarction Pathway among Patients and Health Professionals". Philosophiae Doctor, Norwegian University of Science and Technology, Bårdsgjerde (2022)

patient participation in health services. Our main contribution has been to add frame factors as a new theme related to previous research (Thompson et al. 2007).

2.5.1 *Interaction, Level of Involvement, and Clinical Context*

The three themes of interaction, level of involvement, and clinical context were adopted from Thompson et al. (2007), an integrative approach to patient participation. The results of this meta-ethnography showed that these themes are consistent with Thompson et al.'s (2007) approach. There seems to be a common understanding among patients, family caregivers, and health professionals that patient participation can only be achieved through willingness from health professionals and patients, two-way communication, and trust and respect between the parties. In accordance with the taxonomy of levels of involvement where information-seeking/receptive and information-giving are lower levels of involvement, information was considered as a building block for patient participation in several of the included studies.

A notable finding was the number of studies exploring how patients, family caregivers, and health professionals experienced shared decision-making in different clinical contexts. In Thompson's (2007) taxonomy of levels of involvement, shared decision-making is defined as an important aspect of patient participation, yet he argues that patient participation does not necessarily include the sharing of decisions, as the patients can choose to delegate the decisions to the health professionals. Several of the included studies emphasised challenges in shared decision-making. Both patients and health professionals experienced that in many clinical settings, patients were not able to participate in shared decision-making, due to an acute and life-threatening condition or because they felt that they lacked health literacy. Patients often claimed that they trusted the health professionals and wanted the physicians to make treatment and medical decisions.

2.5.2 Frame Factors

Frame factor theory provides an approach for understanding patient participation processes in a new way that can give insight into what hinders and promotes these processes. Administrative and physical frames, legislation, organisational health literacy, and collaboration will be important frame factors in health services that may promote or hinder patient participation. Administrative and physical frames include access to health professionals, time, and rooms for consultation. Legislation consists of, for example, patient and user rights, clinical guidelines, and standardised clinical pathways. Organisational health literacy is how organisations enable individuals to find, understand, and use information and services to inform health-related decisions and actions (Centers for Disease Control and Prevention (CDC) 2020). To achieve patient participation in clinical pathways, there is a need for collaboration between patients, family caregivers, and health personnel. Findings from this meta-ethnography pinpointed that interprofessional collaboration and coordination between different health professionals and healthcare organisations are important for patient participation. In addition, patients and their family caregivers should be involved in their care and treatment. Collaboration may also be linked to SDG 17, Partnership for goals. Global collaboration through international guidelines and clinical recommendations have been highlighted as important frame factors for quality in care and treatment. Identifying and analysing frame factors in patient participation processes will provide valuable knowledge to strengthen patient participation in practice.

Frame factors are constantly changing and are different depending on the context, however they can provide an open approach to gain new knowledge about patient participation processes. The frame factors do not consist of predetermined variables, but allow an open approach, enabling us to understand and explain various conditions that can promote or hinder patient participation in different clinical pathways or contexts (Kvalsund 1998).

Including frame factors adds a new dimension to the understanding of patient participation. Patient participation is dynamic, complex, and contextual. This qualitative meta-ethnography has shown that frame factors can promote and hinder patient participation. Frame factors have not previously been highlighted in definitions, theoretical approaches, and research on patient participation, and therefore appear to be under-communicated. Frame factor theory may be useful in understanding and revealing the complexity of patient participation in clinical practice and research.

Frame factors provide insight into opportunities and limitations for patient participation in practice. Putting the spotlight on frame factors can contribute to an understanding of how to create sustainable healthcare services. The Shanghai Declaration (WHO 2017) focused on three pillars to achieve the sustainability goals: good governance, healthy cities, and health literacy. A dynamic approach and commitment at the micro, meso, and macro level is necessary to achieve these sustainability goals. Patient participation is closely linked to health literacy, as it empowers patients and enables patient participation.

The comprehensive model will be valuable in developing health professionals' knowledge about patient participation. The model is a useful resource in curricula for bachelor's and master's degrees in nursing, medical education, and other relevant healthcare and social care educations.

2.5.3 *Strengths and Limitations*

A broad systematic search was conducted, and we applied precise inclusion and exclusion criteria to avoid selection bias. We selected studies conducted in middle- and high-income countries to ensure transferability of the findings; 17 of the included studies are from Norway and several of them are authored by the authors of this chapter. This can be both a strength and a weakness. The authors are familiar with the research field, and the majority of the studies were identified in the systematic search.

Most of the studies were conducted in a Nordic context, and this may have an impact on the transferability of the findings to other countries and cultures. In Nordic countries, democratic values, equality, and patient involvement are highly valued and legislated. It is a strength that the analysis is based on empirical studies from countries that have similar healthcare systems.

2.6 Conclusion

There is a lack of research on patient participation in low-income countries. Our comprehensive model for patient participation might be appropriate for studying patient participation in different cultures and healthcare systems. We consider that the four themes in the model are also generally valid and relevant for low-income countries. The content of the themes would be contextual and culturally determined. The model may reveal facilitators and hindrances for the implementation of patient participation and equality globally.

Acknowledgements The authors would like to especially thank Monica Cecilia Marchant, Librarian at the Norwegian University of Science and Technology in Ålesund, for her hard work and help in developing the search strategy and structuring the literature search.

References

Aasen EM, Kvangarsnes M, Heggen K (2012a) Nurses' perceptions of patient participation in hemodialysis treatment. Nurs Ethics 19:419–430. https://doi.org/10.1177/0969733011429015

Aasen EM et al (2012b) The next of kin of older people undergoing haemodialysis: a discursive perspective on perceptions of participation. J Adv Nurs 68:1716–1725. https://doi.org/10.1111/j.1365-2648.2011.05854.x

Aasen EM, Kvangarsnes M, Heggen K (2012c) Perceptions of patient participation amongst elderly patients with end-stage renal disease in a dialysis unit. Scand J Caring Sci 26:61–69. https://doi.org/10.1111/j.1471-6712.2011.00904.x

Andersen-Hollekim T et al (2019) Patient participation in the clinical pathway – nurses' perceptions of adults' involvement in haemodialysis. Nurs Open 6:574–582. https://doi.org/10.1002/nop2.241

Andersen-Hollekim T et al (2020) Narratives of patient participation in the clinical pathway of haemodialysis. J Clin Nurs 29:2293. https://doi.org/10.1111/jocn.15238

Andersen-Hollekim T et al (2021a) Nephrologists' experiences with patient participation when long-term dialysis is required. BMC Nephrol 22:1–10. https://doi.org/10.1186/s12882-021-02261-w

Andersen-Hollekim T et al (2021b) Shared decision-making in standardized cancer patient pathways in Norway – narratives of patient experiences. Health Expect 24:1780–1789. https://doi.org/10.1111/hex.13317

Angel S, Frederiksen KN (2015) Challenges in achieving patient participation: a review of how patient participation is addressed in empirical studies. Int J Nurs Stud 52:1525–1538. https://doi.org/10.1016/j.ijnurstu.2015.04.008

Arnstein SR (1969) A ladder of citizen participation. J Am Plan Assoc 35:216–224. https://doi.org/10.1080/01944366908977225

Ashworth PD, Longmate AM, Morrison P (1992) Patient participation: its meaning and significance in the context of caring. J Adv Nurs 17:1430–1439. https://doi.org/10.1111/j.1365-2648.1992.tb02814.x

Bårdsgjerde EK (2022) Perceptions of patient participation in the myocardial infarction pathway among patients and health professionals. Philosophiae Doctor. Norwegian University of Science and Technology (NTNU)

Bårdsgjerde EK et al (2019) Patient's narratives of their patient participation in the myocardial infarction pathway. J Adv Nurs 75:1063–1073. https://doi.org/10.1111/jan.13931

Bårdsgjerde EK et al (2020) Nurses' perceptions of patient involvement in the myocardial infarction pathway. Nurs Open 7:1606–1615. https://doi.org/10.1002/nop2.544

Bårdsgjerde EK et al (2022) Physicians' perceptions of patient participation in the myocardial infarction pathway. Commun Med. https://doi.org/10.1558/cam.20555

Brownlea A (1987) Participation: myths, realities and prognosis. Soc Sci Med 25:605–614. https://doi.org/10.1016/0277-9536(87)90085-2

Cahill J (1996) Patient participation: a concept analysis. J Adv Nurs 24:561–571. https://doi.org/10.1046/j.1365-2648.1996.22517.x

Cahill J (1998) Patient participation – a review of the literature. J Clin Nurs 7:119–128. https://doi.org/10.1046/j.1365-2702.1998.00132.x

Castro EM et al (2016) Patient empowerment, patient participation and patient-centeredness in hospital care: a concept analysis based on a literature review. Patient Educ Couns 99:1923–1939. https://doi.org/10.1016/j.pec.2016.07.026

Centers for Disease Control and Prevention (CDC) (2020) What is health literacy. Available https://www.cdc.gov/healthliteracy/learn/index.html. Accessed 28 Aug 2023

Christie GP, Ratzan SC (2019) Beyond the bench and bedside: health literacy is fundamental to sustainable health and development. Inf Serv Use 39:79–92. https://doi.org/10.3233/SHTI200061

Cohen E, Botti M (2015) Cancer patients' perceptions of the barriers and facilitators to patient participation in symptom management during an episode of admission. Cancer Nurs 38:458–465. https://doi.org/10.1097/NCC.0000000000000226

Creswell JW (2014) Research design qualitative, quantitative and mixed methods approaches, 4th edn. SAGE, Los Angeles, California

Dahllöf U (1967) Skoldifferentiering och undervisningsførlopp: komparativa mål- och processanalyser av skolsystem I [School differentiation and teaching processes: comparative goal and process analyses of school systems I]. Almqvist & Wiksell, Stockholm

Dahllöf U (1998) En återblick på det tidiga ramfaktorteoretiska tänkandet och några av dess senare utlöpare [A review of the early framework factor theoretical thinking and some of its later offshoots]. In: Kvalsund R et al (eds) I lærande fellesskap [In learning communities]. Høgsulen i Volda og Møreforskning Volda, Volda

France EF et al (2019) Improving reporting of meta-ethnography: the eMERGe reporting guidance. J Adv Nurs 75:1126–1139. https://doi.org/10.1111/jan.13809

Halabi IO et al (2020) 'Patient participation' and related concepts: a scoping review on their dimensional composition. Patient Educ Couns 103:5–14. https://doi.org/10.1016/j.pec.2019.08.001

Höglund AT et al (2010) Patient participation during hospitalization for myocardial infarction: perceptions among patients and personnel. Scand J Caring Sci 24:482–489. https://doi.org/10.1111/j.1471-6712.2009.00738.x

Ibrahim F et al (2019) 'I want to know why and need to be involved in my own care…': a qualitative interview study with liver, bile duct or pancreatic cancer patients about their experiences with involvement in care. Support Care Cancer 27:2561–2567. https://doi.org/10.1007/s00520-018-4548-8

Jerpseth H et al (2018) Older patients with late-stage COPD: their illness experiences and involvement in decision-making regarding mechanical ventilation and noninvasive ventilation. J Clin Nurs 27:582–592. https://doi.org/10.1111/jocn.13925

Kitson A et al (2013) What are the core elements of patient-centred care? A narrative review and synthesis of the literature from health policy, medicine and nursing. J Adv Nurs 69:4–15. https://doi.org/10.1111/j.1365-2648.2012.06064.x

Kvalsund R (1998) Om det konstruerande i utdanningsforskinga [About the constructive in educational research]. In: Kvalsund R et al (eds) I lærande fellesskap [In learning communities]. Høgskulen i Volda og Møreforskning Volda, Volda

Kvangarsnes M et al (2013a) Intensive care unit nurses' perceptions of patient participation in the acute phase of chronic obstructive pulmonary disease exacerbation: an interview study. J Adv Nurs 69:425–434. https://doi.org/10.1111/j.1365-2648.2012.06021.x

Kvangarsnes M et al (2013b) Narratives of breathlessness in chronic obstructive pulmonary disease. J Clin Nurs 22:3062–3070. https://doi.org/10.1111/jocn.12033

Landstad BJ, Kvangarsnes M (2020) Theoretical perspectives and qualitative designs in research on patient participation. Michael 17:181–197

Landstad BJ, Tarberg AS, Kvangarsnes M (2023) Physicians' narratives of communication with patients and their relatives in different phases of the palliative pathway. BMJ Open 13:e065681. https://doi.org/10.1136/bmjopen-2022-065681

Lin C et al (2019) Perceptions of patient participation in symptom management: a qualitative study with cancer patients, doctors, and nurses. J Adv Nurs 75:412–422. https://doi.org/10.1111/jan.13853

Longtin Y et al (2010) Patient participation: current knowledge and applicability to patient safety. Mayo Clin Proc 85:53–62. https://doi.org/10.4065/mcp.2009.0248

Lundgren UP (1972) Frame factors and the teaching process: a contribution to curriculum theory and theory of teaching. Almqvist & Wiksell, Stockholm

Netsey-Afedo MML et al (2020) No time for reflection: patient experiences with treatment-related decision-making in advanced prostate cancer. Scand J Caring Sci 34:880–888. https://doi.org/10.1111/scs.12794

Noblit GW, Hare RD (1988) Meta-ethnography: synthesizing qualitative studies. Sage, London

Orkan O (2019) From Saranac Lake to Shanghai: a brief history of health literacy. In: Orkan O et al (eds) International handbook of health literacy. Policy Press, Bristol

Oxford English Dictionary (2021) Oxford English Dictionary The definitive record of the English language. Oxford University

Sahlsten MJM et al (2008) An analysis of the concept of patient participation. Nurs Forum 43:2–11. https://doi.org/10.1111/j.1744-6198.2008.00090.x

Schildmann J et al (2013) 'One also needs a bit of trust in the doctor…': a qualitative interview study with pancreatic cancer patients about their perceptions and views on information and treatment decision-making. Ann Oncol 24:2444–2449. https://doi.org/10.1093/annonc/mdt193

Sørensen K (2019) Defining health literacy: exploring differences and commonalities. In: Orkan O et al (eds) International handbook of health literacy. Policy Press, Bristol

Svavarsdóttir MH, Sigurðardóttir ÁK, Steinsbekk A (2015) What is a good educator? A qualitative study on the perspective of individuals with coronary heart disease. Eur J Cardiovasc Nurs 15:513–521. https://doi.org/10.1177/1474515115618569

Tarberg AS et al (2019) Silent voices: family caregivers' narratives of involvement in palliative care. Nurs Open 6:1446–1454. https://doi.org/10.1002/nop2.344

Tarberg AS et al (2020) Nurses' experiences of compassionate care in the palliative pathway. J Clin Nurs 29:4818–4826. https://doi.org/10.1111/jocn.15528

Tarberg AS et al (2022) Physicians' perceptions of patient participation and the involvement of family caregivers in the palliative care pathway. Health Expect 25:1945–1953. https://doi.org/10.1111/hex.13551

Thaysen HV, Lomborg K, Seibaek L (2019) Patient involvement in comprehensive, complex cancer surgery: perspectives of patients, relatives and health professionals. Eur J Cancer Care (Engl) 28:e13071. https://doi.org/10.1111/ecc.13071

Thompson A (2007) The meaning of patient involvement and participation in health care consultations: a taxonomy. Soc Sci Med 64:1297–1310. https://doi.org/10.1016/j.socscimed.2006.11.002

Thompson A et al (2007) An integrative approach to patient participation in consultations. In: Collins S et al (eds) Patient participation in health care consultations qualitative perspectives. Open University Press, Maidenhead

Tobiano G et al (2015) Patient participation in nursing care on medical wards: an integrative review. Int J Nurs Stud 52:1107–1120. https://doi.org/10.1016/j.ijnurstu.2015.02.010

Tong A, Sainsbury P, Craig J (2007) Consolidated criteria for reporting qualitative research (COREQ): a 32-item checklist for interviews and focus groups. Int J Qual Health Care 19:349–357. https://doi.org/10.1093/intqhc/mzm042

Vaage S (1998) Perspektivtaking og rammefaktorar [Perspectives and frame factors]. In: Kvalsund R et al (eds) I lærande fellesskap [In learning communities]. Høgskulen i Volda og Møreforskning Volda, Volda

Vahdat S et al (2014) Patient involvement in health care decision making: a review. Iran Red Crescent Med J 16:e12454. https://doi.org/10.5812/ircmj.12454

WHO (1994) A declaration on the promotion of patients' right in Europe. Available https://www.who.int/genomics/public/eu_declaration1994.pdf. Accessed 28 Aug 2023

WHO (2013) Exploring patient participation in reducing health-care-related safety risks. Available https://iris.who.int/bitstream/handle/10665/326442/9789289002943-eng.pdf?sequence=1&isAllowed=y. Accessed 28 Aug 2023

WHO (2017) Shanghai declaration on promoting health in the 2030 Agenda for Sustainable Development. Available https://www.who.int/publications/i/item/WHO-NMH-PND-17.5. Accessed 28 Aug 2023

Wilson T et al (2017) Patient perspectives on engagement in decision-making in early management of non-ST elevation acute coronary syndrome: a qualitative study. BMC Med Inform Decis Mak 17:1–7. https://doi.org/10.1186/s12911-017-0555-9

Årestedt L et al (2019) Patient participation in dialysis care – a qualitative study of patients' and health professionals' perspectives. Health Expect 22:1285. https://doi.org/10.1111/hex.12966

Chapter 3
Using Qualitative Design to Study Health Literacy

Bodil J. Landstad and Marit Kvangarsnes

Abstract Health literacy is critical for mobilising human and societal capital for patients, users, health professionals, organisations, and political bodies. Health reforms and changes in health services require continuous research into how health professionals and organisations can strengthen users' health literacy and sustainable health services. We present qualitative designs which are appropriate for gaining knowledge to strengthen health literacy and to reach the Sustainable Development Goal (SDG 3) which deals with good health and well-being.

Keywords Societal capital · Qualitative design · Social constructivism · Lifeworld · Narrative approach · Hermeneutic circle · Critical discourse

3.1 Background

Health literacy is a complex concept that requires undertaking research from different perspectives and diverse scientific fields. The understanding of diverse perspectives from healthcare providers and patients is vital to build and strengthen health literacy in the population (Rahja et al. 2018). Health literacy is acknowledged globally as important for people's health and well-being, which is one of the UN's Sustainable Development Goals (SDG 3). Health literacy was previously understood as individuals' ability to read, understand, and apply health information to

B. J. Landstad
Department of Health Sciences, Mid Sweden University, Östersund, Sweden

Unit of Research, Education and Development, Östersund Hospital, Östersund, Sweden

M. Kvangarsnes (✉)
Department of Health Sciences in Ålesund, Norwegian University of Science and Technology (NTNU), Ålesund, Norway

Medical Department, Ålesund Hospital, Møre og Romsdal Hospital Trust, Ålesund, Norway
e-mail: marit.kvangarsnes@ntnu.no

T. Hole et al. (eds.), *Towards Sustainable Good Health and Well-being*,
https://doi.org/10.1007/978-3-031-61810-9_3

make healthcare-related decisions (WHO 2013). In 2020, organisational health literacy was also defined as being important. This is the degree to which organisations equitably enable individuals to find, understand, and use information and services in order to inform health-related decisions and actions for both themselves and others (CDC 2020).

The WHO (2013) emphasises that health literacy is both an asset and a form of social capital for individuals and communities. Communities can benefit from their members' health literacy and also have a responsibility to empower people as citizens, members of the workforce, consumers, and patients, so that they can improve their health literacy and thus better make decisions about their health. It has been of concern for many years now that patients with limited health literacy often have difficulties in managing chronic diseases (Keller et al. 2008), lower rate of medication adherences (Berkman et al. 2011; Kripalani et al. 2006), increased emergency care use, and increased risk of hospitalisation (Berkman et al. 2011; Howard et al. 2005; DeWalt et al. 2007).

Countries all over the world have therefore long since recognised the impact of low health literacy on health systems, and considerable efforts are being made to address this. International collaboration, national policy, and legal regulations in this area are some of the steps being taken to reduce the risk of low health literacy (WHO 2013). Research has shown that increased emphasis should be placed on education and training of health professionals in order to improve the practice of health literacy screening and communication (Rahja et al. 2018). Knowledge about health literacy studied from different scientific perspectives is crucial for improving Good health and well-being (SDG 3), Gender equality (SDG 5), Reduced inequalities (SDG 10), and Sustainable cities and communities (SDG 11).

3.2 Qualitative Design

Health professionals who work with health literacy demand evidence-based knowledge at individual and system levels, together with the recognition that health literacy always has a cultural and contextual dimension. Qualitative research, therefore, is relevant when exploring people's experiences with health literacy. Qualitative methods capture the perspective of the individual and their individuality and are used when little is known about a topic or phenomenon (Johnson and Christensen 2016). Qualitative research focuses on analysing the subjective meaning or the social production of issues, events, or practices by collecting data in the form of text or visual materials.

Qualitative inquiry studies interpret how human beings construct and attach meanings to their experiences and, interviews and observations reveal those meanings and their implications (Patton 2015). Qualitative inquiry can illuminate how any human phenomenon unfolds as it does and the effect on those who participate. Stories can be captured to understand people's perspectives and experiences.

Elucidating how systems function and their consequences for peoples' lives is an important aspect of qualitative research and understanding contexts: how and why it matters are also vital. Revealing the intended and unintended consequences of change processes is very important. Qualitative inquiry gives the opportunity to make case comparisons to discover important patterns and themes across cases (Patton 2015). Despite challenges and controversies or criticisms that can arise, knowledge from qualitative research can make a real difference and can address many of the SDGs which aim to improve society and the world at large.

Qualitative design includes both methodology and method. Methodology deals with the underlying theoretical thoughts behind science and philosophical premises for distinct designs such as hermeneutics, phenomenology, narrative inquiry, and critical discourse analysis. Methods deal with specific procedures such as interviews, observations, visual material, and texts used to collect data. Distinct qualitative designs and their underlying thoughts and historical roots are presented in order to illustrate this.

3.3 The Use of Theory in Qualitative Research

As researchers, we have experienced the significance of using theory as an opportunity for making our underlying thoughts and choices visible. The theory is often presented in the background section of a paper and explains the phenomena that will be studied. Furthermore, broader theories often encompass theory which can be applied at distinctive levels, offering methodology, theory, methods, and study topics. Some theories have a clear political aspect, such as critical discourse analysis (Fairclough 1992).

Qualitative researchers may use theory in several ways. (1) It is used as a broad explanation of the phenomenon being studied, for example, a social constructivist approach might be used to study learning (Wenger 2004). The primary focus of this theory is learning as social participation (Wenger 2004). (2) Theoretical lenses or perspectives provide an overall approach for the research questions being posed. These lenses, in some designs, become a transformative perspective that shapes the types of research questions, inform how data are collected and analysed, and suggest a call for action (Creswell and Creswell 2018). (3) Qualitative theory may be the endpoint of a study (Glaser and Strauss 1967). Shaping theory is a process which necessitates many steps. First, the researcher decides how to collect data through, for example, interviews or observations. Researchers then ask participants open-ended questions or write fieldnotes. Third, the researcher analyses data in order to form patterns or themes. Finally, the researcher creates theories from the data and literature which has been appraised. Some qualitative studies, however, do not use any explicit theory, e.g. phenomenology. The aim is to build the essence of experience from participants (Patton 2015). Creswell and Creswell (2018) give some advice on the use of theory in qualitative research:

1. Decide if theory is to be used in the research.
2. Identify how the theory will be used, as a transformative advocacy lens, an up-front explanation, or as an end point.
3. Locate the theory early or at the end.

Most qualitative analyses start with an inductive approach which is a bottom-up perspective, while a deductive approach is a top-down perspective. Inductive analyses bring you from the specific to the general, while deductive analyses bring you from the general to the specific. Most qualitative analyses are inductive as well as deductive. The researcher often starts from the raw data to identify topics before returning to the raw data to see how the various main topics are corroborated by the material (Creswell and Creswell 2018).

3.4 Studying Health Literacy: A Range of Qualitative Designs

The qualitative designs presented in Table 3.1 give an overview of distinct designs that can be used in qualitative research to illuminate different dimensions of health literacy. We have chosen to present various designs that we have used in our own studies, and that are mostly used in studying health literacy. Other qualitative designs might have the potential to illuminate various aspects of the importance of health literacy.

3.4.1 *Phenomenological Perspective*

The purpose of a phenomenological approach is to illuminate the essence of peoples' lived experiences related to a particular phenomenon (Patton 2015). Phenomenology is especially relevant when studying patients' lived experiences with illness. This methodology will give insights into the patient's lived experience of the illness and their health literacy. In the phenomenological tradition, rich and thick data are collected to give valuable insights when working on strengthening patients' health literacy.

The world in which we live, and with which we have immediate familiarity and experience, is in phenomenology called the *lifeworld* (Husserl 1965). Husserl argues that knowledge has a validity regardless of when, and by whom, it is formulated. The world can be nothing else than the world as it appears in our consciousness. The concept, *lifeworld*, does not consider power relationships in society, i.e. social conflicts and conflicts of interest between diverse groups (Crossley 1996).

The phenomenological inquiry framework has developed over time and its key contributors are Schütz (1899–1959), Merleau-Ponty (1908–1961), Whitehead (1861–1947), and Giorgi (1931–). Patton points to the fact that, over time, phenomenology has become so widely embraced that its meaning has become unclear

Table 3.1 Major features of distinct qualitative designs

Qualitative design	Purpose	Data collection methods	Analyses	Study objects	Dimensions of health literacy
Phenomenology	To uncover what a particular experience means to a group of people and how they experienced it	Individual interviews Focus group Participant observation Personal text	Analysis of the essence of lived experiences. The experiences of different people are bracketed, analysed, and compared to identify the essence of the phenomenon	Patients, relatives, health professionals	Uncovering the essence of lived experience of illness
Narrative	To understand people's lives through first-person stories	Narrative interviews Documents/texts (letters, diaries)	The analyses explore lived experiences through a focus on personal narratives, revealing aspects of lives previously hidden from social science	Patients, relatives, health professionals	Deeper understanding of how social factors affect people's opportunities to make healthy choices
Hermeneutics	To interpret texts on health literacy in historical and cultural contexts	Individual interviews Focus groups Observations Documents/texts	Hermeneutic interpretation of text – Using the hermeneutic circle; understanding the part and the whole through iterative recontextualisation	Patients, relatives, health professionals, health policy processes	To interpret health literacy in a historical and cultural context
Grounded theory	To develop alternative theories based on the context in which the phenomenon has arisen	A fundamental principle is that 'all is data'—For example, Individual interviews Focus groups Observations Documents/texts (letters, speeches, memoirs, novels, biographies, newspaper articles) Visual expressions (photographs, films) Websites	The analysis is based on observations rather than using analytical constructs, categories or variables from already proposed or established theories	Patients, relatives, health professionals, health policy processes	Building alternative theories on health literacy

(continued)

Table 3.1 (continued)

Qualitative design	Purpose	Data collection methods	Analyses	Study objects	Dimensions of health literacy
Social constructivism	To understand how health literacy is developed in different settings	Individual interviews Focus group Observations Documents/texts Websites Visual expressions (pictures)	Social constructivist analysis—Meaning is created in social interactions	Patients, relatives, health professionals, health policy processes	Understanding health literacy on individual and societal levels
Critical discourse analysis	To analyse underlying power structures in communication	Individual interviews Focus group Observations Documents/texts Websites	Analysis at three levels: Text Discursive practice Social context	Patients, relatives, health professionals, health policy processes	To identify witch discourses that dominate communication in health literacy

(Patton 2015). The key element of a phenomenological research study is that the researcher attempts to understand how people experience a phenomenon from each person's own perspective. The aim is to enter the inner world of each participant in order to understand his or her perspective or experience (Johnson and Christensen 2016). This is a high ambition, and we question if this is possible to achieve.

Phenomenology might serve as a relevant research approach when studying patients' experiences of treatment in critical and life-threatening situations. Torheim and Kvangarsnes (2014) explored patient experiences with chronic obstructive pulmonary disease exacerbation and mask treatment. The study created an understanding of patients' vulnerability during interaction and involvement with health professionals in acute treatment of chronic obstructive pulmonary disease. This knowledge is important for health personnel when helping patients cope with mask treatment in a life-threatening situation.

Knowledge about patient experiences is important when facilitating individual learning processes. Uncovering the essence of the lived experience of illness and treatment in different phases is vital when planning, implementing, and assessing person-centred learning processes for good health and well-being.

3.4.2 Narrative Approach

Using a narrative approach is a way of gaining a greater understanding of patients' experiences and may contribute to knowledge that can provide more effective care and treatment (Holloway and Freshwater 2007). The word 'narrative' comes from Latin 'narrate' which means to tell a story. A story usually features a series of events. A narrative approach to studying patients gives them both a clear voice and attributes them with significance. By highlighting patients' own perceptions around participation, health professionals can gain a new understanding of the patient's situation, and patients', as well as relatives' health literacy (Chase 2018).

Narrative analysis includes a theoretical direction that captures personal and human dimensions of experience over time which considers the relationship between individual experience and cultural context (Clandinin and Connelly 2000). Narrative analysis provides an alternative to the understanding of the individual as *abstracted* out of his or her context rather than being a part of it (Holloway and Freshwater 2007).

There are various understandings of what narrative research includes, and the definition of the word 'narrative' itself has changed over time. Chase (2018) describes the development from which narrative was exclusively used to illuminate the past and present, to inclusion of the future, in narrative presentations. A narrative approach is appropriate when studying health literacy in a clinical pathway. When including the future within a narrative, it can potentially provide an insight into how to improve health literacy for patients and their families.

The selection of informants for narrative research is often strategic: it aims to capture the complexity of health literacy. Shaping the narrative might be built on experiences not only from one patient but also from several (Brinkmann and Kvale 2015). When you have several informants, the interviews are presented as one narrative, which represents an interpretation of all the patients' stories. The narrative is also created with the help of documents describing the context of the research, diaries, and information about the researcher's role as a *research tool*.

In narrative analysis one searches for a plot, which is a pattern of developments in the stories. The plot may, for example, describe health literacy in distinct phases of a patient pathway (Holloway and Freshwater 2007; Patton 2015). Important topics in narrative research are (1) the theoretical framework on which the study is based, (2) the type of knowledge to which the personal narratives give us access (3) the ethical position the researcher holds in the presentation of data, and (4) the methods that should be used to produce narrative data (Thomas 2010). Explicitness about the underlying choices taken is important for the credibility of narrative research (Chase 2018).

During the last decade, narrative inquiry is moving towards theoretical and methodological maturity (Chase 2018). To elucidate the thoughts underpinning such a study, the reader should be provided with information that may furnish a deeper understanding of the findings and the opportunity to make their own judgement of the trustworthiness of the study (Patton 2015).

Narrative approaches have proven invaluable in illuminating both the patients' and relatives' experiences of health literacy (Tarberg et al. 2019; Bårdsgjerde et al. 2019). Family caregivers in palliative care have experienced low health literacy in that they were not prepared for the terminal phase of their beloved family members (Tarberg et al. 2019). Health literacy and patient participation differed throughout various phases of the myocardial infarction pathway (Bårdsgjerde et al. 2019). This study showed that health literacy needed to be improved on both individual and organisational levels. Narratives give the informants a clear voice and offer access to subjective experiences that can provide a deeper understanding of their health literacy. Chapter 9 is an example of how the narrative approach gives new knowledge on how the visually impaired experience education and learning from a lifespan perspective.

3.4.3 Hermeneutic Approach

Hermeneutics is the theory and methodology of interpretation. Etymologically, the word comes from the ancient Greek *hermeneuein*, which means 'to express', in the sense of conveying and speaking. The word is threefold: to express, to interpret, and to translate (Gulddal and Møller 1999).

Hermeneutics has developed since ancient times, and dialogue is held up as an ideal for understanding and knowledge development. Philosophers such as Schleiermacher (1758–1834), Dilthey (1833–1911), Heidegger (1889–1976), Gadamer (1900–2002), and sociologists such as Habermas (1929) and Ricoeur (1913–2005) have been central in the development of hermeneutics into a philosophy of understanding (Gulddal and Møller 1999). Hermeneutics is the most important theory of science in the humanities.

The *hermeneutic circle* is a key concept and refers to the idea that the understanding of a text is based on the understanding of each, distinct, individual part. Interpretation is a process that oscillates between parts and the overall context in which the part exists. Prejudice is part of the human horizon of understanding and is, as such, an important gateway to interpretation and understanding (Gadamer 1999). The challenge is to separate valid prejudices from those which are invalid. This must be examined in relation to how one previously looked at a case. The interpreter's pre-understanding must be examined by time intervals, changed, and adjusted in the light of new experiences. The time interval often makes it possible to solve the critical questions of hermeneutics, the separation of the true prejudices that make us understand from the false ones that make us misunderstand (Gadamer 1999; Gulddal and Møller 1999).

Gadamer's texts on understanding have later been criticised, nuanced, and problematised by, for instance, Habermas (1999). A hermeneutic understanding is developed by the interpreter listening to the text and asking questions in order to interpret the underlying meaning. The text must be interpreted in its historical and cultural context and read with empathy. The art is to bring out what is not present in the text (Marquard 1999).

Alvesson and Sköldberg (2009) emphasise the following underlying principles in hermeneutic research:

1. Interpretation should have a logical context.
2. Overview of the totality of the work.
3. Underlying problems must emerge.
4. All the questions that the text raises must be answered.
5. The questions must come from the text and not from the interpreter.
6. The text must be interpreted in a historical and cultural context.
7. The interpreter must respect what the author says.
8. The interpreter must respect established interpretations of text.
9. The interpretation must stimulate further thinking.
10. The interpretation can be transferred to other areas.

Different hermeneutic traditions may be perceived as being incompatible (Gilje 2019); however, various traditions can provide complementary understanding in interpreting the data. Different approaches can be united in a specific research project and benefit from each other. A hermeneutic approach was used in a study of children and adolescents' mental health during the Covid-19 pandemic in Canada (Montreuil et al. 2022). Repercussions of social isolation were a central finding. The participants in the study experienced loneliness and a longing to be with their peers. Coping strategies reported were having a variety of hobbies, expressing their emotions, and accessing financial and material resources. The interviews were analysed following a narrative synthesis approach, through which the experiences were contrasted and contextualised to highlight relevant themes. The study emphasised the importance of supporting children's and adolescents' mental health during a pandemic. The study is relevant for clinical practice and policy improvement, in particular in finding means for social engagement whilst maintaining safety (Montreuil et al. 2022).

The above example gives important knowledge for providing good health and well-being for children during times of crises such as a pandemic. Hermeneutic design is relevant when we wish to interpret the complexity in the human dimensions. This is important knowledge when health professionals are planning comprehensive and health-literate learning processes that also include mental health.

3.4.4 Grounded Theory

Grounded theory can be considered both as a qualitative design and as a method for developing new and context-specific theories (Starrin 1996). The theory is a suitable method for studying social processes such as user participation and health literacy in health services (Foley and Timonen 2015; Charmaz et al. 2018).

Glaser and Strauss (1967) developed a systematic method containing both qualitative and quantitative elements that allow data to be moved to theory (induction) to create alternative theories. Such theories will be related to the context in which they are developed. The foundation of grounded theory is based on observations rather than on predefined analytical constructs, categories, or variables from already established theories. The theory emerges from a substantial field of research as documented by Starrin and Svensson in their work (1996). Prominent phases or concepts in grounded theory are (Willig 2013):

1. Categories (groupings of cases).
2. Coding (the categories are identified).
3. Constant comparative analysis (identification of similarities and dissimilarities between categories).
4. Negative case analysis (development of theory considering current evidence).
5. Theoretical sensitivity (from a descriptive to analytical level).
6. Theoretical sampling (collecting additional data based on categories that have emerged in previous phases of the analysis).
7. Theoretical saturation (samples and encodes data until new categories cease to apply).
8. Memo writing (written record containing the theory development).

Glaser and Strauss (1967) assumed that everyone could create their own theory, if it is based on real life, and they believed that everyone can be innovative in social research, as so-called *science entrepreneurs*.

Grounded theory has, for instance, been used in cardiovascular research (Dunn Margaritis & Anderson 2017). This study investigated patients' and health personnel's perspectives on how health literacy skills were developed in patients with cardiovascular disease or diabetes. The study revealed that social support,

Internet searches, personalised instructional strategies, and self-directed learning were important. Social support was found to be a key factor in developing health literacy skills (Dunn et al. 2017). An article using grounded theory (Landstad et al. 2022) found that participating in peer-led self-help groups can assist with the transfer of learning to new environments, including increased work capacity.

Grounded theory has been used in many research projects to highlight health literacy at individual and organisational levels. Grounded theory is an appropriate design to use when we know very little about a phenomenon and prefer an inductive approach.

3.4.5 Social Constructivist Approach

Social constructivism points to the fact that the individual is socially constructed through interactions with others. This perspective is promising in research on health literacy. It has the potential to highlight the cultural dimension in developing health literacy at individual and organisational levels.

Social constructivism is a broad approach and is challenging to define. Howitt (2010) presents four characteristics of social constructivism:

1. Historical and cultural specificity of knowledge.
2. Critical position towards *taken for granted knowledge.*
3. Knowledge sustained by social interactions.
4. Knowledge and social interactions integrated.

A fundamental understanding in social constructivism is that all human cognition is socially constructed (Berger and Luckmann 2000; Mead et al. 2015). Knowledge is a result of the development of culture, and the historical and contemporary context of within which the individual is a part (Howell 2013). The various fields in social constructivism are rooted in pedagogy, sociology, linguistics, philosophy, and the social sciences. This interdisciplinary approach has gained significant importance in many academic environments and has contributed to theory development.

Patton (2015) has proposed the use of core elements of the social construction inquiry framework, some of which are of specific relevance when studying health literacy. Based on these, we have formulated areas important to illuminate in a social constructivist perspective. The significance of understanding multiple realities within, and between, groups of patients in order to facilitate different learning processes is crucial. Cultural competence is required in contact with different patient groups. Language and how a message is communicated is also important to study. Digitalisation of the healthcare sector will give patients different access to health services depending on digital competence. We have little knowledge about how the lack of digital competence affects people's health. Research on how power differentials affect and shape social interactions and perceptions of health services may provide important knowledge for building equal access to health services.

A study from Southwest China shows that the digital health literacy level of community-dwelling older adults is relatively low, with the need to be improved urgently (Liu et al. 2022). The European Health Literacy Population Survey (2019–2021) indicates limited health literacy in large groups of the general population in all countries but to varying degrees depending on the country (WHO 2021). There were vulnerable sub-populations in all countries, for instance, senior citizens, low education, financial difficulties, low self-assessed social status, low self-assessed health status, and frequent user of healthcare services. There is a lack of knowledge about how people can develop digital health skills in order to maintain good health and well-being (SDG 3).

Social constructivism can give insight in vulnerable sub-population participation in digital learning processes in communities of practices (Wenger 2004). Social constructivism is focusing on learning as an inherently and social process that cannot be separated from the social context in which it happens. This perspective can give insight into how participating in communities of practices may lead to health-literate processes or outbound trajectories. Learning means participating in communities of practices in a way that the person becomes digitally health literate.

3.4.6 Critical Discourse Analysis

Critical discourse analysis aims at uncovering implicit power structures in texts by using linguistic analyses linked to the historical and social contexts of which the texts are a part. The aim of these analyses is to create change and contribute to democracy, freedom, and equality (Fairclough 1992, 2001).

This theoretical approach focuses on how language works in maintaining and change power relations in society (Fairclough 2001). Studies of language can reveal these processes and focus on how people can become more conscious of them, and more able to resist and change them.

By performing in-depth text analyses and considering the social and historical context in which the text is included, this approach allows one to emphasise how society's hierarchies of power are created and reproduced through discursive practice.

Patient participation is intricately linked to health literacy and concerns the distribution of power between patients and health professionals (Thompson 2007). Critical discourse analysis may provide insights into how the patient's right to participation is safeguarded in various levels and contexts. Globally, the right of patients to participate in treatment has been strengthened (WHO 2013). The WHO suggests that users should be involved in the shaping of all parts of the health service. It is important to study how legislation on patient participation and legislation on health literacy is implemented in clinical work both at a system level and in the formulation of national guidelines for treatment. Earlier research has shown disappointing results (Røsvik et al. 2010). Apart from very few exceptions, patients had not participated in developing the guidelines examined.

Critical discourse analysis is based on a discursive event, which is the use of language in a specific situation (Fairclough 1992). Analyses at three levels are carried out: (1) text analysis (for example, wording, sentence level, and modalities), (2) discursive practice (production of text, distribution processes, and how a text is consumed), and (3) discourse as social practice: ideology and hegemony (discourse is placed in an understanding of power at the system level).

Critical discourse analysis involves analysing the relationship between text, interaction, and context (Fairclough 1992). Several researchers have been inspired by linguist Fairclough when studying patient participation in clinical activities in acute and chronic diseases (Aasen et al. 2012a; Kvangarsnes et al. 2013). These studies show the benefit of combining text analysis and analysis of discursive practice with theoretical models of patient participation. The studies highlight ethical dilemmas in treatment in both acute and chronic situations. Linguistic analyses uncover power structures and lack of participation in health services (Aasen et al. 2012b; Kvangarsnes et al. 2013). Contradictions are uncovered between the rhetoric in health policy documents and the experiences of patients and health professionals with patient participation.

Empowering the patient to make good choices for their good health and well-being is emphasised internationally (WHO 2013). However, important hidden obstacles still exist. In such cases, critical discourse analyses may provide valuable insights for changing and building equity in access to health services.

Using critical discourse analysis can be useful for uncovering how health literacy is addressed at the micro, meso, and macro levels in health services. By connecting the various levels, it is possible to gain an increased understanding of the discourse on health literacy in society.

3.5 Data Collection in Qualitative Research on Health Literacy

Health literacy can be studied from the perspectives of patients, relatives, or health professionals. Research shows that patients and health professionals may experience health services differently (Sahlsten et al. 2007). There are various data collection methods for studying health literacy.

Interviews are often semi-structured or narrative. In semi-structured interviews, an interview guide with various topics one wishes to illuminate is used. A theoretical framework on health literacy can, for example, provide suggestions for themes in an interview guide. Knowledge of patient experiences may provide new insights for use in the development of health services and medical guidelines (Røsvik et al. 2010).

Health professionals' experiences might be illuminated through focus groups, in order to acquire rich data. A homogeneous group is recommended because they have a common frame of reference for discussions (Krueger and Casey 2015). Experience has shown that homogeneous groups are suitable for producing complex experiences and ethical dilemmas in healthcare (Tritter and Landstad 2020). In heterogeneous groups, various positions, and different frames of reference, may hinder deeper communication of the phenomenon being studied (Tritter and Landstad 2020).

Observation could be another method employed for studying health literacy. Different observation methods are available: participatory, systematic, or video recording (Patton 2015). An ethical dilemma associated with the observation of patients, however, is that a patient being observed may find it stressful to have a researcher present during treatment.

Document and text analysis is a method that can be used to provide insight into how health professionals communicate with patients and relatives (Bratberg 2017). Table 3.1 presents examples of documents and texts which are relevant to such analysis.

Photovoice is a method that can be used to document and reflect the health literacy of diverse groups to add knowledge that is intended to create change (Wang and Burris 1997). The participants are given the task of documenting their situation with the help of visual narratives. Photovoice can be helpful in revealing how patients experience their situation.

3.6 Qualitative Design, Health Literacy, and Sustainable Development Goals

Qualitative design presents insights into humans' experiences of health, illness, health literacy, and health services. This is important knowledge that can provide understanding as to what might facilitate, and what might hinder, attaining SDGs.

The study of different texts and political documents has the potential to reveal underlying and hidden power structures that can hinder empowering people and providing equity in society. Different qualitative designs provide opportunities for diverse types of knowledge and partly overlap in terms of their focus.

To study health literacy from either an individual level, a phenomenological perspective, narrative approach, or grounded theory may be a question of making an appropriate choice. Knowledge of any patient's subjective experience of illness and their situation will be important for health professionals so that they can strengthen health literacy and adapt it to that individual's needs. All these perspectives highlight the importance of the user's voice and may additionally be used as a resource for eradicating poverty which is one of the most important sustainability goals (SDG1). To study patients' clinical pathways from the perspective of patients and family caregivers may provide new insights for shaping sustainable health services for good health and well-being.

Social constructivism and hermeneutic approaches are relevant when studying health literacy in social settings, i.e. when seeking to explore how societal, historical, local, pragmatic, and other factors influence the construction or interpretation of knowledge about health literacy.

To study health literacy at an organisational level, a social constructivist and hermeneutic perspective will offer insight into interactions between health professionals and patients. Patients' and users' access to health services will be a key area to study when considering how to achieve relevant sustainability goals. A critical discourse analysis may uncover underlying power structures in communication between patients and the system, which may provide insights for building equality, which is also fundamental in attaining any relevant sustainability goals such as Good health and well-being (SDG 3), Gender equality (SDG 5), Reduced inequalities (SDG 10), and Sustainable cities and communities (SDG 11).

References

Aasen EM, Kvangarsnes M, Heggen K (2012a) Nurses' perceptions of patient participation in hemodialysis treatment. Nurs Ethics 19:419–430

Aasen EM, Kvangarsnes M, Heggen K (2012b) Perceptions of patient participation amongst elderly patients with end-stage renal disease in a dialysis unit. Scand J Caring Sci 26:61–69

Alvesson M, Sköldberg K (2009) Reflexive methodology: new vistas for qualitative research. Sage, London

Bårdsgjerde EK, Kvangarsnes M, Landstad BJ et al (2019) Patient's narratives of their patient participation in the myocardial infarction pathway. J Adv Nurs 75(5):1063–1073. https://doi.org/10.1111/jan.13931

Berger PL, Luckmann T (2000) The social construction of reality: a treatise in the sociology of knowledge. Penguin Books Ltd, London

Berkman ND, Sheridan SL, Donahue KE et al (2011) Low health literacy and health outcomes: an updated systematic review. Ann Intern Med 155(2):97–107

Bratberg Ø (2017) Tekstanalyse for samfunnsvitere [text analysis for social scientists]. Cappelen Damm akademisk, Oslo

Brinkmann S, Kvale S (2015) InterViews: learning the craft of qualitative research interviewing. Sage, Thousand Oaks

CDC- Centers for Disease Control and Prevention (2020) What is health literacy? Retrieved from https://www.cdc.gov/healthliteracy/learn/index.html

Charmaz K, Thornberg R, Keane E (2018) Evolving grounded theory and social justice inquiry. In: Denzin NK, Lincoln YS (eds) The Sage handbook of qualitative research, 5th edn. Sage, Los Angeles

Chase SE (2018) Narrative inquiry toward theoretical and methodological maturity. In: Denzin NK, Lincoln YS (eds) The Sage handbook of qualitative research, 5th edn. Sage, Los Angeles

Clandinin DJ, Connelly FM (2000) Narrative inquiry: experience and story in qualitative research. Jossey-Bass, San Francisco

Creswell JW, Creswell JD (2018) Research design: qualitative, quantitative & mixed methods approaches. Sage, Los Angeles

Crossley N (1996) Intersubjectivity: the fabric of social becoming. Sage, London

DeWalt DA, Dilling MH, Rosenthal MS et al (2007) Low parental literacy is associated with worse asthma care measures in children. Ambul Pediatr 7(1):25–31

Dunn PJ, Margaritis V, Anderson CL (2017) Use of grounded theory in cardiovascular research. Qual Rep 22(1):197–212. Retrieved from http://nsuworks.nova.edu/tqr/vol22/iss1/11
Fairclough N (1992) Discourse and social change. Polity Press, Cambridge
Fairclough N (2001) Language and power. Longman, Harlow
Foley G, Timonen V (2015) Using grounded theory method to capture and analyze health care experiences. Health Serv Res 50:1195–1210
Gadamer H (1999) Forståelens historicitet som hermeneutisk princip [The historicity of understanding as a hermeneutic principle]. In: Gulddal J, Møller M (eds) Hermeneutik: en antologi om forståelse [Hermeneutics: an anthology of understanding]. Gyldendal, København
Gilje N (2019) Hermeneutikk som metode: ein historisk introduksjon [Hermeneutics as a method: a historical introduction]. Samlaget, Oslo
Glaser BG, Strauss AL (1967) The discovery of grounded theory: strategies for qualitative research, vol 17. Aldine de Gruyter, New York, p 364
Gulddal J, Møller M (1999) Hermeneutik: en antologi om forståelse. Gyldendal, København
Habermas J (1999) Kraften i de bedre argumenter [The power of better arguments]. Ad notam Gyldendal, Oslo
Holloway I, Freshwater H (2007) Narrative research in nursing. Blackwell, Oxford
Howard DH, Gazmararian J, Parker RM (2005) The impact of low health literacy on the medical costs of Medicare managed care enrollees. Am J Med 118(4):371–377
Howitt D (2010) Introduction to qualitative methods in pshycology. Person Education Limited, Essex
Husserl E (1965) Philosophy as rigorous science. In: Husserl E (ed) Phenomenology and the crisis of philosophy. Philosophy as rigorous science and philosophy and the crisis of European man. Harper & Row, New York
Johnson RB, Christensen L (2016) Educational research. Quantitative, qualitative, and mixed approaches, 6th edn, Thousand Oak, Sage
Keller DL, Wright J, Pace HA (2008) Impact of health literacy on health outcomes in ambulatory care patients: a systematic review. Ann Pharmacother 42(9):1272–1281
Kripalani S, Henderson LE, Chiu EY et al (2006) Predictors of medication self-management skill in a low-literacy population. J Gen Intern Med 21(8):852–856
Krueger RA, Casey MA (2015) Focus groups: a practical guide for applied research. Sage, Los Angeles
Kvangarsnes M, Torheim H, Hole T et al (2013) Intensive care unit nurses' perceptions of patient participation in the acute phase of chronic obstructive pulmonary disease exacerbation: an interview study. J Adv Nurs 69:425–434
Landstad BJ, Hedlund M, Kendall E (2022) Practicing in a person-centred environment. Self-help groups in psycho-social rehabilitation. Disabil Rehabil 44(7):1067–1076. https://doi.org/10.1080/09638288.2020.1789897
Liu SZ et al (2022) Current status and influencing factors of digital health literacy among community-dwelling older adults in Southwest China: a cross-sectional study. BMC Public Health 22:996. https://doi.org/10.1186/s12889-022-13378-4
Marquard O (1999) Spørgsmålet om det spørgsmål, som hermeneutikken er svar på [The question of the question to which hermeneutics is the answer]. In: Gulddal J, Møller M (eds) *Hermeneutik: en antologi om forståelse* [Hermeneutics: an anthology of understanding]. Gyldendal, København
Mead GH, Morris CW, Huebner DR et al (2015) Mind, self, and society. University of Chicago Press, Chicago/London
Montreuil M, Gendron-Cloutier L, Laberge-Perrault E, Piché G, Genest C, Rassy J, Malboeuf-Hurtubise C, Gilbert E, Bogossian A, Camden C, Mastine T, Barbo G (2022) Children and adolescents' mental health during the COVID-19 pandemic: a qualitative study of their experiences. J Child Adolesc Psychiatr Nurs 1–10:65. https://doi.org/10.1111/jcap.12404
Patton MQ (2015) Qualitative research & evaluation methods: integrating theory and practice. Sage, Los Angeles

Rahja R, Hassali MAA, Jou LC, Murugiah MK (2018) The perspective of healthcare providers and patients on health literacy: a systematic review of the quantitative and qualitative studies. Perspect Public Health 138:2. https://doi.org/10.1177/1757913917733775

Røsvik AH, Movik E, Nylenna M (2010) Deltar pasientene i utviklingen av kliniske retningslinjer i Norge? [Do patients participate in the development of clinical guidelines in Norway?]. Tidsskr Nor Laegeforen 130:2236–2238

Sahlsten MJ, Larsson IE, Sjöström B et al (2007) Patient participation in nursing care: towards a concept clarification from a nurse perspective. J Clin Nurs 16:630–637

Starrin B (1996) Grounded theory – En modell för kvalitativ analys [A model for qualitative analysis]. In: Starrin B, Svensson P-G (eds) Kvalitativa studier i teori och praktik [Qualitative studies in theory and practice]. Lund, Studentlitteratur

Starrin B, Svensson P-G (1996) Kvalitativa studier i teori och praktik. Studentlitteratur, Lund

Tarberg AS, Kvangarsnes M, Hole T, Tronæs M, Landstad BJ (2019) Silent voices: family caregivers' narratives of involvement in palliative care. Nurs Open 6:1446–1454

Thomas C (2010) Negotiating the contested terrain of narrative methods in illness contexts. Sociol Health Illn 32:647–660

Thompson A (2007) The meaning of patient involvement and participation in health care consultations: a taxonomy. Soc Sci Med 64:1297–1310

Torheim H, Kvangarsnes M (2014) How do patients with exacerbated chronic obstructive pulmonary disease experience care in the intensive care unit? Scand J Caring Sci 28:741–748

Tritter J, Landstad BJ (2020) Focus groups. In: Mays N, Pope C (eds) Qualitative research in health care, 4th edn. Blackwell BMJ Books, Malden, pp 57–66

Wang C, Burris MA (1997) Photovoice: concept, methodology, and use for participatory needs assessment. Health Educ Behav 24:369–387

Wenger E (2004) Knowledge management as a doughnut: shaping your knowledge strategy through communities of practice. Ivey Business Journal 2004:1

WHO (2013) Kickbusch, I, Pelikan JM, Apfel F, Tsouros AD (eds) Health Literacy. The solid facts. https://apps.who.int/iris/bitstream/handle/10665/128703/e96854.pdf

WHO (2021) Short summary of the international report on the methodology, results, and recommendations of the European Health Literacy Population Survey 2019–2021 (HLS19) of M-POHL. Available https://m-pohl.net/sites/m-pohl.net/files/inline-files/HLS19%20Short%20Summary.pdf. Accessed 24 Feb 2024

Willig C (2013) Introducing qualitative research in psychology. McGraw-Hill Education, Maidenhead

Part II
Pedagogical Approaches to Building Health Literacy

Chapter 4
Building Health Literacy: A Pedagogical Model for Good Health and Well-Being

Marit Kvangarsnes, Torstein Hole, Bodil J. Landstad, Berit Misund Dahl, and Elise Kvalsund Bårdsgjerde

Abstract The aim of this chapter is to present a pedagogical model for building health literacy to obtain sustainable health services at both an individual and organisational level. Health-literate people and organisations are better able to access, analyse, and comprehend necessary health information to make appropriate decisions about health and well-being. Promoting health literacy is a priority for the World Health Organization, and lack of health literacy is a global concern. Health literacy is important for health promotion and disease prevention and is particularly significant for people with chronic diseases. Health professionals need pedagogical knowledge and tools to build health literacy and to promote good health and well-being, which is an important Sustainability Development Goal (SDG 3).

M. Kvangarsnes (✉)
Department of Health Sciences in Ålesund, Norwegian University of Science and Technology (NTNU), Ålesund, Norway

Medical Department, Ålesund Hospital, Møre og Romsdal Hospital Trust, Ålesund, Norway
e-mail: marit.kvangarsnes@ntnu.no

T. Hole
Medical Department, Ålesund Hospital, Møre og Romsdal Hospital Trust, Ålesund, Norway

Faculty of Medicine and Health Sciences, Norwegian University of Science and Technology (NTNU), Trondheim, Norway

B. J. Landstad
Department of Health Sciences, Mid Sweden University, Östersund, Sweden

Unit of Research, Education and Development, Östersund Hospital, Östersund, Sweden

B. M. Dahl
Department of Health Sciences, Norwegian University of Science and Technology, Ålesund, Norway

Department of Public Health, University of Stavanger, Stavanger, Norway

E. K. Bårdsgjerde
Department of Health Sciences in Ålesund, Norwegian University of Science and Technology (NTNU), Ålesund, Norway

T. Hole et al. (eds.), *Towards Sustainable Good Health and Well-being*,
https://doi.org/10.1007/978-3-031-61810-9_4

A pedagogical model offers a systematic and universal approach for planning, implementing, and assessing health literacy. Moreover, the pedagogical model for health literacy is a useful tool for reaching sustainability goals related to good health and well-being and better opportunities for all. The model aims at liberating human resources and promoting equity and consists of six pedagogical categories: frame factors, content, goals, patients' health literacy, communication, and assessment. The pedagogical model has an ecological approach. This means that individuals, social networks, organisations, communities, and population must be engaged in order to build health literacy. Educational interventions also play a vital role in building health literacy, such as schools which have a focus on promoting good health. Building health literacy needs to start in early childhood and span over an individual's lifetime.

Keywords Health literacy · Pedagogic · Sustainability · Learning · Pedagogical model · Health education

4.1 Introduction

Health literacy is key to achieving sustainability in healthcare services. The Shanghai Declaration (WHO 2017) highlighted that health literacy involves more than just providing information and health education: it also involves enabling people to gain access to, understand, and use information in a way that promotes good health and well-being for themselves, their families, and the society, thus leading to a healthier population globally.

The understanding of health literacy has developed over time (Parnell 2015). In 1998, the World Health Organization (WHO) defined health literacy as follows:

> Cognitive and social skills which determine the motivation and ability of individuals to gain access to, understand and use information in ways which promote and maintain good health. (WHO 1998)

The definition describes health literacy at an individual level, but the term is equally important at an organisational level. Organisational health literacy may concern how easy organisations make it to navigate, understand, and use information and services (Brach et al. 2012; Brega et al. 2019; Bremer et al. 2021). Brega et al. (2019) highlight three key areas for strengthening health literacy at an organisational level: (1) communication, (2) conditions for navigating health services, and (3) individually adapted services and practice communities that offer a learning environment that promotes health literacy. A shift in the understanding of health literacy has been described. Parnell (2015) claims that health literacy is about the relationship between the skills of persons receiving care or treatment and the professionals or systems that are providing the care and treatment. In 2020, Centers for Disease Control and Prevention (CDC) presented the following definitions for personal and organisational health literacy:

"*Personal health literacy* is the degree to which individuals have the ability to find, understand, and use information and services to inform health-related decisions and actions for themselves and others"
"*Organizational health literacy* is the degree to which organizations equitably enable individuals to find, understand, and use information and services to inform health-related decisions and actions for themselves and others"

These definitions both emphasise the individuals' ability to use health information and make "well-informed" decisions and acknowledge the organisations' responsibility in addressing and incorporating health literacy in health services (Centers for Disease Control and Prevention (CDC) 2020).

People's health literacy and participation in health services change over time and are contextual (Thompson 2007; Ministry of Health and Care Services 2019; Bårdsgjerde 2022; Kvangarsnes et al. 2023). Studies show that people with high health literacy are better equipped to participate in decisions about care and treatment that affect one's life (WHO 2016b; Ministry of Health and Care Services 2019).

In order to strengthen the population's health literacy, public health nurses and health professionals should be working with preventive and therapeutic health measures (WHO 2013a, 2023; Ministry of Health and Care Services 2019). Health education to increase health literacy worldwide is a priority for the WHO, and lack of health literacy is a global concern (WHO 2013a, 2016a; Dietscher et al. 2019). Health literacy is important in health promotion, disease prevention, adherence to treatment, and is particularly significant for people with chronic diseases (WHO 2016a; Ministry of Health and Care Services 2019; The Norwegian Directorate of Health 2020). Efforts to strengthen health literacy among the population require commitments at various levels (Brach et al. 2012; Sørensen et al. 2012, 2021; WHO 2013a).

The aim of this study is to develop a pedagogical model for building health literacy, leading to good health and well-being based on a narrative review (Baethge et al. 2019). Health literacy is a vital asset for promoting good health and well-being, corresponding to the UN Sustainability Development Goal (SDG) 3. The pedagogical model is universal, and globally relevant, serving as a supportive tool for promoting equality and quality in education which are important aspects for sustainable development. The 2030 Agenda for Sustainable Development reflects the complexity and interconnectedness of equality and quality (WHO 2017). It considers widening economic and social inequalities, rapid urbanisation, threats to the climate and the environment, burden of infectious diseases, and emerging challenges such as non-communicable diseases.

4.2 Design and Methods

This study employs qualitative design and is based on a narrative review (Creswell and Creswell 2018; Baethge et al. 2019). Traditionally, a narrative review is a comprehensive, critical, and objective analysis and synthesis of the current knowledge on a topic. In this study, a narrative review has been conducted to identify, map, and synthesise earlier pedagogical models, research with relevance, and the researchers' knowledge and experiences, to develop a universal model for pedagogical work to improve health literacy (Baethge et al. 2019).

The narrative review was conducted using the steps set out by Baethge et al. (2019):

1	Justification of the study. This is carried out in the introduction.
2	Aim clearly stated. The present study aimed at developing a pedagogical model for building health literacy.
3	Description of the literature search. First, we searched for pedagogical models for planning, implementing, and evaluating education. In particular, we have further developed an established pedagogical model, *the didactic relationship model* (Bjørndal and Lieberg 1978). Second, we searched for literature in Oria, which is a Norwegian library database containing international books, electronic books, research articles, journals, and electronic documents. Our educational and research background was important when mapping relevant literature and research in developing the pedagogical model. Communication and health pedagogy is considered important in national strategies to increase health literacy in the population, as mentioned earlier in this chapter (WHO 2013a; Ministry of Health and Care Services 2019). Whilst conducting the literature search, we searched for research on communication, health literacy, and patient participation in health services to substantiate the model.
4	Key statements throughout the article are supported by relevant and updated references.
5	Scientific reasoning. The development of the model is based on a comprehensive literature review. The synthesis of the literature led to a universal model illuminating the complexity of health literacy. We have selected literature from various fields to shed light on the challenges and the complexity of building health literacy in health services.
6	Presentation of data. The didactic relationship model has for years been used at various levels of the Norwegian education system. We have developed this model for new areas, and combined knowledge from different fields to customise it when building health literacy is the goal of the learning process. In addition, our model is underpinned by medical and healthcare research that provides insight into the special challenges in the field of healthcare to enhance health literacy and sustainability. Theories of didactics, ethics, patients, and health professionals' experiences of learning processes and patient participation in health services became important sources.

We labelled six categories relevant for the universal pedagogical model for good health and well-being: *frame factors, content, goals, patients' health literacy, communication*, and *assessment*, based on the review and discussions in the research group. The labelled categories have different content in various contexts.

Finally, health professionals analyse, synthesise, and describe the categories in the model in relation to their unique situation. The model should not be used prescriptively, but as a tool for reflection in which the essentials in each pedagogical situation are considered. The research group consisted of researchers with backgrounds in pedagogical, medical, nursing, and social sciences. Knowledge from various fields was important to adapt the model to healthcare contexts.

4.3 Pedagogical Models

The pedagogical model is developed from the didactic relationship model (Kvangarsnes et al. 2023). The didactic relationship model was originally developed for primary schools (Bjørndal and Lieberg 1978) but has been adopted across other levels of education. Tyler's *Basic principles of curriculum and instruction* (Tyler 1949) provides the backdrop for understanding the development of the didactic relationship model.

4.3.1 Tyler's Basic Principles of Curriculum and Instruction

Ralph Tyler's model deals with ways to formulate, organise, and evaluate educational objectives. Tyler (1949) and his ideas have had a major influence not only across all levels of schools but also in society at large (Martinsen 2005; Martinsen 2006). The model is based on causality, an underlying belief that an action will lead to a predictable result. Four fundamental questions for planning teaching were important in this model:

1. What educational objectives should the school seek to attain?
2. What educational experiences can be provided that are likely to achieve these objectives?
3. How can these educational experiences be effectively organised?
4. How can we determine whether these objectives are achieved? (Tyler 1949)

This model presents learning as a linear process that takes place in various stages. Criticism gradually grew against the measure/means thinking both in pedagogy and in health sciences (Stenhouse 1975; Eisner 1985; Martinsen and Wærness 1991). One counterargument was that educational actions cannot be reduced to technique and that learning is far more complex. Understanding learning in a cause/effect framework is, among other things, criticised for being too simplistic and instrumental. Teaching technology was criticised because the human dimension of teaching disappeared. Self-instructive material was criticised because the programme provided little contact between teacher and student and among the students. There was also a concern that knowledge might be reduced to fields that can be measured and controlled. Requirements for measurable knowledge may mean that attitudinal and qualitative knowledge may be given less status and emphasis (Stenhouse 1975; Eisner 1985; Kvangarsnes et al. 2023).

4.3.2 The Didactic Relationship Model

The development of the didactic relationship model was an attempt to create an alternative approach to the measure/means model to clarify the interaction between key factors that influence the learning situation (Bjørndal and Lieberg 1978). The model was a Norwegian contribution to create a comprehensive model for planning teaching or learning and was designed after the authors had experienced that strong goal management training did not work in practice. One of the goals of didactic relation thinking was to promote learning as a creative process. There was a desire to develop a model to give thinking and action patterns grounded in attitudes and values that could contribute to a positive and open learning process in which those involved participated and assumed responsibility for their learning (Kvangarsnes et al. 2023). The didactic relationship model consists of six didactic categories: goals, content, participant assumptions, assessment, working methods, and frame factors. All categories are equally important. There is also a logical connection between the distinct categories, which affect each other mutually. The overall objective provides direction for the educational reflections, planning, and implementation of the learning process (Bjørndal and Lieberg 1978).

4.4 A Pedagogical Model for Good Health and Well-Being

Based on the narrative review, we developed a pedagogical model for building health literacy and good health and well-being (Fig. 4.1). A similar model for building health literacy has been presented by the authors in a Norwegian textbook for public health nurses (Kvangarsnes et al. 2023). This model has been expanded and adapted to sustainable good health and well-being. Five features characterise this model:

1. The purpose of the model is to provide a comprehensive and universal pedagogical approach to plan, implement, and assess learning processes to build health literacy and sustainable health services at individual, group, population, and organisational levels.
2. The model consists of six pedagogical categories. We analyse and synthesise several categories in the situation and then develop and design learning processes.
3. The six pedagogical categories are frame factors, content, goals, patients' health literacy, communication, and assessment. All of these are interrelated.
4. The model invites a systematic and comprehensive approach in educational work: each situation is unique.
5. The model should be understood within an ecological perspective (Sørensen et al. 2012). People gain health literacy depending on the social and the cultural contexts in which they are living. This means that a wide range of learning opportunities should be offered. Interactions within and between the various contexts will be significant. For example, cooperation between family and school will be important for a child's learning of health literacy.

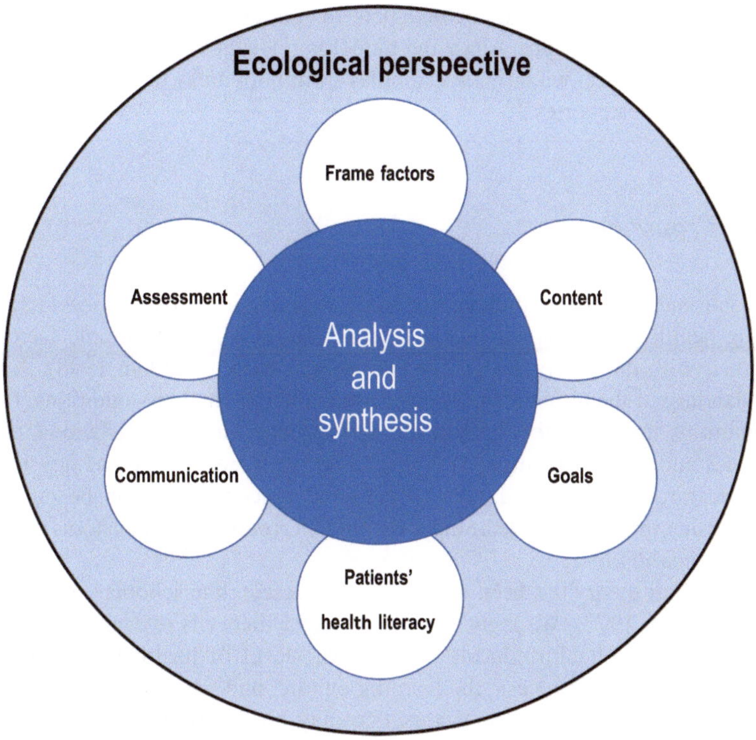

Fig. 4.1 A Pedagogical model for good health and well-being. (Author's own figure. Modified from Kvangarsnes et al. 2023)

This pedagogical model is a valuable tool in mapping important elements that are valid in learning situations when the goal is to strengthen health literacy. Health professionals need to map the content of the pedagogical categories in every unique situation and be aware of how the different categories are interrelated and impact each other. Using this model will contribute to professionalism and awareness in health professionals' pedagogical work in various phases of the patient's learning process. By analysing and synthesising the didactic categories as well as designing a pedagogical program for each unique situation, health professionals will ensure quality in the learning processes for the patients. This model is useful for reaching several of the sustainability goals. It can help to strengthen good health and well-being for patients (SDG 3) at the same time as being a tool for health professionals to ensure quality in work to strengthen patients' health literacy (SDG 4). The model's underlying idea is to liberate the patients' resources and contribute to equity in health services (SDG 1).

Reflections related to the six pedagogical categories are explained in more detail in the following paragraphs. Since the model is relevant for preventive and therapeutic health services, we provide examples from both areas in the presentation of the pedagogical categories.

4.4.1 Frame Factors

Organisational structures, policy, and leadership are important frame factors for building health literacy at the macro level (Brega et al. 2019). Frame factors are concerned with the preconditions for educational work (Gundem 1998). A broad understanding of the term encompasses formal and informal preconditions. Formal preconditions in the context of a health service may include legislations, clinical guidelines and checklists, time, as well as learning materials such as physical and digital resources (Bårdsgjerde 2022). Informal preconditions can be defined as usual practice in a hospital, learning environment, routines, and customs related to promoting health literacy.

Frame factor theory has been used to conduct research in schools (Dahllöf 1967, 1998; Lundgren 1972). We argue that frame factor theory is relevant for analysing and understanding health education work. The level of health literacy of those involved in a learning process, the learning culture, and the culture of cooperation between professions are frame factors that may either promote or inhibit health education work (Kvangarsnes et al. 2023). The organisation of a health service may also prove to be relevant frame factors. At an organisational level, communication, conditions for navigating health services, and individually adapted services and practice communities offering a learning environment that promotes health literacy have proven to be significant frame factors (Brega et al. 2019).

Fragmented health services can result in a lack of continuity (Bårdsgjerde 2022) which has unfortunate consequences on the learning process. Bårdsgjerde (2022) found that frame factors in relation to how the patient pathway for acute myocardial infarction was organised, prevented continuity of information and involvement at a patient level.

Studies have highlighted the importance of creating health literate–friendly organisations aiming to strengthen patients' health literacy and participation in treatment and care (Andersen-Hollekim et al. 2021; Tarberg et al. 2022). In a study, nephrologists suggested that patients requiring dialysis could learn how to cannulate their fistula, set up the machine, and run the dialysis session themselves (Andersen-Hollekim et al. 2021). Another example of health literate–friendly organisations is applying advanced care plans (ACP) in palliative care. Physicians considered ACP as a tool for open and good dialogue including patient and family caregiver's future expectations and their thoughts regarding participation in treatment and care (Tarberg et al. 2022).

The right of patients and their next of kin to information and participation is embedded in legislation. It has been demonstrated that acute situations reduce the need for participation (Thompson 2007; Bårdsgjerde et al. 2019; Kvangarsnes et al. 2020). In chronic diseases, on the other hand, it is vitally important that the patient is involved in treatment decisions (Thompson 2007; Landstad et al. 2020). There is considerable variation in the need for information and participation for different patient groups and in distinct phases of a patient pathway. The WHO has promoted a person-centred approach to the patient, emphasising the importance of user involvement and equality (WHO 2013b).

4.4.2 *Content and Goals*

Health professionals are expected to consider participants' prerequisites according to content and goals (Act related to patients' rights 1999, last changed 2020). Different situations require various levels of information and participation, and people have a range of preferences and needs (Kvangarsnes et al. 2023). Age, earlier experience, life stage, sociocultural, and linguistic background are all examples of prerequisites that are important in educational work.

It is essential that health professionals have reliable professional knowledge. Knowledge of disease, treatment, medication, and how to prevent any infection or complications of disease or treatment is vital. For chronic diseases, it will be valuable that the patient obtains knowledge about the reference range for blood tests and other parameters, enabling them to take responsibility for observing any potential development of the disease. To reduce the mortality of non-communicable diseases, such knowledge is necessary for prevention as well as secondary prevention.

Knowledge is an important fundament for building health literacy and can be classified at distinct levels. In the 1950s, a classification system was developed for learning goals in three areas: cognitive goals (knowledge), affective goals (attitudes and values), and psychomotor goals (skills). The classification of knowledge measures developed by the American psychologist Benjamin Bloom (1956) is the most commonly used taxonomy, where knowledge is divided into six hierarchically ordered classes (Fig. 4.2).

Assessing the level of knowledge that is desirable for each patient, group, and situation is crucial. All users/patients are different, and coping with diseases requires health-literate patients who understand the consequences of the different choices available to them. Formulating personalised goals is imperative. This requires continuous dialogue with users and their relatives. For some patients, it is important to assess blood test values or other parameters to be able to dose insulin, heart medicine, or painkillers. This necessitates that the patient or user holds the necessary knowledge about specific situations and can then apply this knowledge in practice. This requires not only a high-level of health literacy but also that the patient or user can analyse different choices in relation to their good health and well-being (Kvangarsnes et al. 2023).

At an individual level, health professionals and users need to cooperate in formulating goals. It is vital that health professionals, patients, and next of kin have

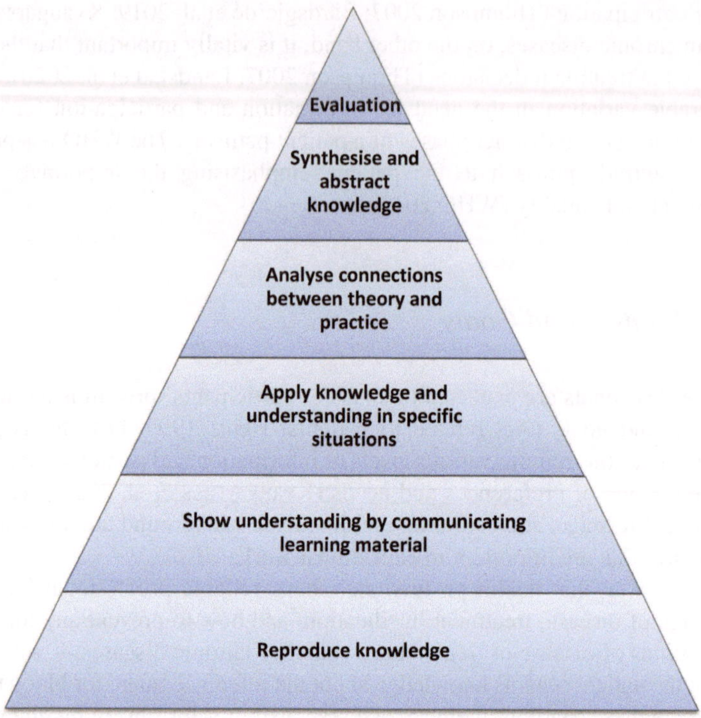

Fig. 4.2 Authors' own figure, based on Bloom's Taxonomy (Bloom 1956)

realistic and coherent goals. A mutual understanding of such goals and a joint point of departure constitute beneficial conditions for positive interaction (Kvangarsnes et al. 2023). Especially in person-centred care, the change in direction from asking "What's the matter?" to "What is important to you?" has been used in the development of coherent patient pathways. The purpose of the question is to obtain information about the patient's preferences, needs, and wishes in relation to health services and the design of the service (Barry and Edgman-Levitan 2012; Oksavik et al. 2020). It may be beneficial to formulate both long-term and short-term goals. This can facilitate a step-by-step and personalised process.

As an example, public health nurses provide teaching and supervision in primary and secondary school on issues concerning sexual health, relationships, lifestyle, and substance abuse, which are critical issues for good health and well-being. Teaching and guidance take place both in groups and individually. These are areas that have elements of knowledge, skills, and values, and yet the topics are very personal. Age, gender, background, and health literacy have an impact on how pupils perceive supervision on such topics (Kvangarsnes et al. 2023). Many individuals may experience shame or believe that public health nurses are intervening in what is considered to be an 'intimate zone' (Gulbrandsen 2006). This may cause the person to withdraw and not take part in a planned session. When it comes to the development of attitudes and values, it is vitally important that the persons are engaged and involved from the planning stage. Pupils could then contribute relevant inputs to the goals and content of the teaching, the potential learning methods, and assessment(s) of the process.

4.4.3 Patients' Health Literacy

Adapting the model for diverse groups requires knowledge about different life phases, functional ability, developmental stages, cultures, and clinical pathways, in addition to basic pedagogical competence (Act related to patients' rights 1999, last changed 2020; Ministry of Health and Care Services 2019). Visual impairment, hearing, or reduced cognitive functions can be a hindrance during work which is striving to strengthen health literacy (Kvangarsnes et al. 2023). Health professionals must be familiar with various technical aids and resources that can ease communication and learning. For example, the National Library in Norway offers audiobooks, non-fiction, newspapers, and journals for people with difficulties in reading printed text and ordinary books due to disability or illness (The Norwegian Library of Talking Books and Braille (NLB) 2022).

The timing of providing information is also essential. Patients who are seriously and acutely ill may not be receptive to information and may only need brief, but precise, communication. Research has shown that, for example, the rehabilitation phase can be a good time for more involvement and building health literacy (Thompson 2007; Bårdsgjerde et al. 2019). Choosing the right time for sharing information is important to build health literacy and ensure good health and promote well-being in a sustainable way. Patients must be at a receptive stage to be able to absorb, assess, and use the information to make appropriate choices according to their health and well-being.

4.4.4 Communication

The word 'communication' comes from the Latin verb *communicare* which means to make common, or share. This is also the goal of health education (Kvangarsnes et al. 2023). Health professionals have a message that they wish to convey, and they hope to create a common frame of reference with an individual or a defined target group. At the same time, the user has experiences, as well as other knowledge, which they can share, which is relevant to healthcare professionals. Communication, therefore, must be a two-way process characterised by dialogue (Madssen 2007). This dialogue will assume different forms depending on the context.

Patient education is often provided in the context of groups set up for that purpose (Kvangarsnes et al. 2023). Cardiac rehabilitation is an example of patient education provided to patients with cardiovascular disease with an emphasis on physical activity through group training, patient education, and individual guidance. Research has shown that cardiac rehabilitation has a positive effect on good health and well-being and reduces risk factors for disease development through increasing health literacy (Rauch et al. 2016; Peersen et al. 2017; Valaker et al. 2017).

At an individual level, health education tends to take the form of supervision. As an example, breastfeeding supervision may help to achieve many of the SDGs such as reducing poverty, hunger, increased health education, gender equality, and sustainable consumption (UNICEF 2016). Increasing breastfeeding rates is clearly important across the globe. Public health nurses are responsible for supervising families undertaking breastfeeding: they meet the mother and the child in intimate and vulnerable situations. The mother has to have confidence in their public health nurse, which means that the mother leaves it to the nurse to give advice that is significant to the child's health (Grimen 2009). This creates a relationship of power, where the trust-giver (mother) is dependent on the competence of the nurse giving access to other supplementary health services. Public health nurses will be dependent on the mother's trust to gain access to knowledge from the mother that supplies the conditions for making good judgement-based decisions. Trust eases the transfer of information and knowledge. If the mother distrusts the nurse, it is likely that relevant information will be withheld. When it comes to caring for infants, this can have fatal consequences. Trust in such health supervision is fundamental to successful outcomes (Kvangarsnes et al. 2023).

Digital development is rapidly transforming the way in which the communication and healthcare information is exchanged together with the volume of information available (Pagliari 2021). This was clearly demonstrated during the outbreak of COVID-19. The use of digital tools and digitalisation has impacted society, and it affects the way we communicate, the pace at which we communicate, and the quantity of information available. This also applies to the health and care services. Digital health services require users to have digital health literacy or electronic health literacy (e-health literacy). This includes everything from searching for, finding, understanding, assessing, and applying health information from electronic sources to be able to apply the knowledge to address or solve a medical problem (Norman and Skinner 2006). E-health literacy in the population can actually create greater inequalities between patient groups in relation to skills and access to health services (Olsson et al. 2019; Kokkinakis 2022). This is an unintended consequence of well-meaning progress.

A Norwegian population survey, which was undertaken as part of The International Health Literacy Population Survey 2019–2022, shows that a substantial proportion of the population is in fact well prepared to use digital health services (The Norwegian Directorate of Health 2020). The same survey also shows that some groups in society report having weaker digital skills, especially older people over the age of 65, immigrants, people with long-term illnesses, and people with low level of education (The Norwegian Directorate of Health 2020, 2021). The concept of digital exclusion in relation to health services is a well-recognised topic in the public debate on the digitalisation of health services (Olsson et al. 2019; Kokkinakis 2022).

Another important issue to consider when addressing communication between health professionals/health organisation and patients/users is to employ language which is accessible, without professional terms that can impede its understanding. Much of the information available is characterised by bureaucratic and a very formal language, often dominated by professional terms (Ministry of Health and Care Services 2019; Hem and Nylenna 2021).

4.4.5 *Assessment*

A distinction is often made between summative and formative assessment (Lauvås and Handal 2014). Summative assessment has a control function and is conducted at the end of a process. In the health services' domain, collecting patient-reported data is common practice. Patient-reported data is information that patients and users themselves report about their own experience related to health and well-being and how satisfied they are with treatment and health services they have encountered. The overall goal in collecting this type of data is to improve the quality of treatment provision (National Service for Medical Quality Registers 2022). Research on patient experiences in different clinical pathways will provide an important knowledge base for health professionals in their efforts to strengthen health literacy. Formative assessment takes place during a learning process. Formative assessment is the most important form of evaluation of health education because it is possible to create a personalised educational process where one can change learning methods, pace, content, and frameworks in accordance with the user's preferences and feedback (Kvangarsnes et al. 2023).

Assessment of health education should take place both during the process as well as at the end. Everyone involved should take part: the knowledge can be used systematically for improvement. Feedback from users and next of kin can be particularly valuable (Kvangarsnes et al. 2023).

In a global and regional context, particularly, the considerable amount of data following the SDG3 is valuable for assessments of good health and well-being for all. The number of indicators has increased from 115 to 217 over the last 6 years (United Nations 2022). This database might give politicians valuable knowledge to prioritise vulnerable groups in the work to strengthen health literacy. 'Leaving no one behind' is an important principle in the SDG goals (United Nations 2022).

4.5 Pedagogical Analysis and Synthesis

The aim behind this universal pedagogical model is to provide health professionals with a model that is relevant in the planning, implementation, and assessment of health pedagogical work to build health literacy. Each situation is unique, and an educational tool that is open, not predetermined and includes significant pedagogical elements, will be valuable for health professionals.

Evidence-based practice must be the starting point for health professionals in designing teaching. Evidence-based practice requires that professional decisions are based on the best available research, along with clinical experience and patients' preferences and needs in each situation. User knowledge and user participation in all phases of the process will be fundamental to pedagogical health work. From time to time, conflict can arise between clinical guidelines and a patient's preferences. It may be the case that patients do not want to receive the recommended medical treatment: this, in turn, may cause ethical dilemmas for health professionals. The principle of autonomy versus beneficence creates challenges in interactions between patient and health professionals (Beauchamp and Childress 2019). Awareness of ethical dilemmas in educational work is vital when safeguarding patients' interests.

Finally, health professionals must synthesise pedagogical categories in the learning process. This may lead to a systematic, conscious, and professionally grounded approach in planning, implementation, and assessment of the learning process. The synthesis aims to create a new understanding of the complexity of the learning process.

4.6 Conclusion and Implications for Practice

We have developed a pedagogical model that could be used as a universal model for supporting health professionals in planning, implementing, and assessing health education at all ages. Patients' preferences and personal values must always be considered and given due respect. Improving health literacy in the population also calls for an ecological perspective when ensuring good health and well-being (Orkan et al. 2019).

The model can support innovation in health services by improving individual and organisational health literacy according to SDG9 (industry, innovation, and infrastructure). A common framework will provide opportunities for strengthening cooperation and communication on health literacy globally. The model has categories that are valid in all learning processes regarding health literacy. Implications for practice are as follows:

- Individuals, social networks, organisations, communities, and population must be included in improving health literacy.
- Schools should promote health literacy within their curricula, and in teaching and learning processes.
- Collaboration between educational systems and health services globally is crucial.
- The pedagogical model can be employed by students, health professionals, social personnel, teachers, health managers, and politicians in improving health literacy globally.

References

Act related to patients' rights (1999, last changed 2020) Lov om pasient- og brukerrettigheter Available https://lovdata.no/dokument/NL/lov/1999-07-02-63. Accessed 28 Aug 2023

Andersen-Hollekim T et al (2021) Nephrologists' experiences with patient participation when long-term dialysis is required. BMC Nephrol 22:1–10. https://doi.org/10.1186/s12882-021-02261-w

Baethge C, Goldbeck-Wood S, Mertens S (2019) SANRA – a scale for the quality assessment of narrative review articles. Res Integr Peer Rev 4:1–7. https://doi.org/10.1186/s41073-019-0064-8

Bårdsgjerde EK (2022) Perceptions of patient participation in the myocardial infarction pathway among patients and healthcare professionals. Philosophiae Doctor. Norwegian University of Science and Technology (NTNU). https://hdl.handle.net/11250/2982645

Bårdsgjerde EK et al (2019) Patient's narratives of their patient participation in the myocardial infarction pathway. J Adv Nurs 75:1063–1073. https://doi.org/10.1111/jan.13931

Barry MJ, Edgman-Levitan S (2012) Shared decision making – the pinnacle patient-centered care. N Engl J Med 9:780–781. https://doi.org/10.1056/NEJMp1109283

Beauchamp TL, Childress JF (2019) Principles of biomedical ethics, 8th edn. Oxford University Press, New York

Bjørndal B, Lieberg S (1978) Nye veier i didaktikken?: en innføring i didaktiske emner og begreper [Breaking fresh ground in didactics?: an introduction to didactical themes and terms]. Aschehoug, Oslo

Bloom B (1956) Taxonomy of educational objectives – the classification of educational goals. Longman, London

Brach C et al (2012) Ten attributes of health literate health care organizations. NAM Perspect. https://doi.org/10.31478/201206a

Brega AG et al (2019) Organizational health literacy: quality improvement measures with expert consensus. Health Lit Res Pract 3:e127–e146. https://doi.org/10.3928/24748307-20190503-01

Bremer D et al (2021) Which criteria characterize a health literate health care organization?–a scoping review on organizational health literacy. BMC Health Serv Res 21:1–14. https://doi.org/10.1186/s12913-021-06604-z

Centers for Disease Control and Prevention (CDC) (2020) What is health literacy. Available https://www.cdc.gov/healthliteracy/learn/index.html. Accessed 28 Aug 2023

Creswell JW, Creswell JD (2018) Research design: qualitative, quantitative & mixed methods approaches, 5th edn. Sage, Los Angeles

Dahllöf U (1967) Skoldifferentiering och undervisningsførlopp: komparativa mål- och processanalyser av skolsystem I [School differentiation and teaching processes: comparative goal and process analyses of school systems I]. Almqvist & Wiksell, Stockholm

Dahllöf U (1998) En återblick på det tidiga ramfaktorteoretiska tänkandet och några av dess senare utlöpare [A review of the early framework factor theoretical thinking and some of its later offshoots]. In: Kvalsund R et al (eds) I lærande fellesskap [In learning communities]. Høgsulen i Volda og Møreforskning Volda, Volda

Dietscher C et al (2019) The Action Network on Measuring Population and Organizational Health Literacy (M-POHL): a network under the umbrella of the WHO European Health Information Initiative (EHII). Public Health Panorama 5:65–71

Eisner E (1985) The art of educational evaluation. A personal view. The Falmer Press, London

Grimen H (2009) Hva er tillit? [What is trust?]. Universitetsforlaget, Oslo

Gulbrandsen P (2006) Skam i det medisinske rom [Shame in the medical room]. Gyldendal akademisk, Oslo

Gundem BB (1998) Skolens oppgave og innhold: en studiebok i didaktikk [The school's task and content: a study book in didactics], 4th edn. Universitetsforlaget, Oslo

Hem E, Nylenna M (2021) Språk er også medisin [Language is also medicine]. Michael 18:7–13

Kokkinakis D (2022) eHealth literacy and capability in the context of the pandemic crisis. In: Erhag HF et al (eds) A multidisciplinary approach to capability in age and ageing. Springer, Cham
Kvangarsnes M et al (2020) Patient participation in acute illness – a metasynthesis of the experiences of patients and health professionals. Michael 17:77–93
Kvangarsnes M, Dahl BM, Bårdsgjerde EK (2023) Helsekompetanse – en pedagogisk modell [Health literacy – a pedagocial model]. In: Dahl BM, Bjørnsen HN (eds) Helsesykepleie i praksis [Public health nursing in practice]. Fagbokforlaget, Bergen
Landstad BJ, Bårdsgjerde EK, Kvangarsnes M (2020) Patient participation in chronic disease – a metasynthesis. Michael 17:95–109
Lauvås P, Handal G (2014) Veiledning og praktisk yrkesteori [Supervision and practical vocational theory], 3rd edn. Cappelen Damm akademisk, Oslo
Lundgren UP (1972) Frame factors and the teaching process: a contribution to curriculum theory and theory of teaching. Almqvist & Wiksell, Stockholm
Madssen K-A (2007) Språk og kommunikasjon: Myndiggjering eller umyndiggjering? [Language and communication: empowerment or disempowerment?]. In: Ekeland T-J, Heggen K (eds) Mesitring og myndiggjering – reform eller retorikk? [Coping and empowerment – reform or rhetoric?]. Gyldendal Akademisk, Oslo
Martinsen K (2005) Samtalen, skjønnet og evidensen [Dialogue, judgement and evidence]. Akribe, Oslo
Martinsen K (2006) Care and vulnerability. Akribe, Oslo
Martinsen K, Wærness K (1991) Pleie uten omsorg? Norsk sykepleie mellom pasient og profesjon [Care without care? Norwegian nursing between patient and profession]. Pax, Oslo
Ministry of Health and Care Services (2019) Strategi for å øke helsekompetansen i befolkningen 2019–2023 [Strategy to increase health literacy in the population 2019–2023]. Availabe https://www.regjeringen.no/contentassets/97bb7d5c2dbf46be91c9df38a4c94183/strategi-helsekompetanse-uu.pdf. Accessed 28 Aug 2023
National service for medical quality registers (2022) Pasientrapporterte data [Patient reported data]. Available https://www.kvalitetsregistre.no/pasientrapporterte-data. Accessed 13 Nov 2023
Norman CD, Skinner HA (2006) eHealth literacy: essential skills for consumer health in a networked world. J Med Internet Res 8:e506. https://doi.org/10.2196/jmir.8.2.e9
Oksavik JD et al (2020) Sharing responsibility: municipal health professionals' approaches to goal setting with older patients with multi-morbidity–a grounded theory study. BMC Health Serv Res 20:1–11. https://doi.org/10.1186/s12913-020-4983-3
Olsson T, Samuelsson U, Viscovi D (2019) At risk of exclusion? Degrees of ICT access and literacy among senior citizens. Inf Commun Soc 22:55–72. https://doi.org/10.1080/1369118X.2017.1355007
Orkan O et al (2019) Introduction. In: Orkan O et al (eds) International handbook of health literacy: research, practice and policy across the lifespan. Policy Press, Bristol
Pagliari C (2021) Digital health and primary care: past, pandemic and prospects. J Glob Health 11. https://doi.org/10.7189/jogh.11.01005
Parnell TA (2015) Health literacy in nursing: providing person-centered care. Springer, New York
Peersen K et al (2017) The role of cardiac rehabilitation in secondary prevention after coronary events. EJPC 24:1360–1368. https://doi.org/10.1177/2047487317719355
Rauch B et al (2016) The prognostic effect of cardiac rehabilitation in the era of acute revascularisation and statin therapy: a systematic review and meta-analysis of randomized and non-randomized studies–The Cardiac Rehabilitation Outcome Study (CROS). EJPC 23:1914–1939. https://doi.org/10.1177/2047487316671181
Sørensen K et al (2012) Health literacy and public health: a systematic review and integration of definitions and models. BMC Public Health 12:1–13. https://doi.org/10.1186/1471-2458-12-80
Sørensen K et al (2021) Building health literacy system capacity: a framework for health literate systems. Health Promot Int 36:i13–i23. https://doi.org/10.1093/heapro/daab153

Stenhouse L (1975) An introduction to curriculum research and development. Heinemann, London
Tarberg AS et al (2022) Physicians' perceptions of patient participation and the involvement of family caregivers in the palliative care pathway. Health Expect 25:1945–1953. https://doi.org/10.1111/hex.13551
The Norwegian Directorate of Health (2020) Befolkningens helsekompetanse, del 1 [Health literacy in the Norwegian population, part 1]. Available https://www.helsedirektoratet.no/rapporter/befolkningens-helsekompetanse/Befolkningens%20helsekompetanse%20-%20del%20I.pdf/_/attachment/inline/e256f137-3799-446d-afef-24e57de16f2d:646b6f5ddafac96eef5f5ad602aeb1bc518eabc3/Befolkningens%20helsekompetanse%20-%20del%20I.pdf. Accessed 28 Aug 2023
The Norwegian Directorate of Health (2021) Helsekompetanse i fem utvalgte innvandrerpopulasjoner i Norge: Pakistan, Polen, Somalia, Tyrkia og Vietnam. Befolkningens helsekompetanse, del II [Health literacy in five selected immigrant populations in Norway: Pakistan, Poland, Somalia, Turkey and Vietnam. The Norwegian population's health literacy, part II]. Available https://www.helsedirektoratet.no/rapporter/befolkningens-helsekompetanse/Befolkningens%20helsekompetanse%20del%20II%20-%20Helsekompetansen%20i%20fem%20utvalgte%20innvandrerpopulasjoner%20i%20Norge.pdf/_/attachment/inline/10dec1b9-0d63-4746-ac27-041ed77238d0:372387142688ef9e57d78ba0f9b4a2f708f40746/Befolkningens%20helsekompetanse%20del%20II%20-%20Helsekompetansen%20i%20fem%20utvalgte%20innvandrerpopulasjoner%20i%20Norge.pdf. Accessed 28 Aug 2023
The Norwegian Library of Talking Books and Braille (NLB) (2022) Available https://www.nlb.no/eng. Accessed 28 Aug 2023.
Thompson A (2007) The meaning of patient involvement and participation in health care consultations: a taxonomy. Soc Sci Med 64:1297–1310. https://doi.org/10.1016/j.socscimed.2006.11.002
Tyler RW (1949) Basic principles of curriculum and instruction. University of Chicago Press, Chicago
UNICEF (2016) Breastfeeding and the Sustainable Development Goals. Available https://worldbreastfeedingweek.org/2016/pdf/BreastfeedingandSDGsMessaging%20WBW2016%20Shared.pdf. Accessed 28 Aug 2023
United Nations (2022) The Sustainable Development Goals Report 2022. Available https://unstats.un.org/sdgs/report/2022/The-Sustainable-Development-Goals-Report-2022.pdf. Accessed 28 Aug 2023
Valaker I et al (2017) Continuity of care after percutaneous coronary intervention: the patient's perspective across secondary and primary care settings. Eur J Cardiovasc Nurs 16:444–452. https://doi.org/10.1177/1474515117690298
WHO (1998) Health promotion glossary. Available https://www.who.int/healthpromotion/about/HPR%20Glossary%201998.pdf?ua=1. Accessed 28 Aug 2023
WHO (2013a) Health literacy The solid facts. Available https://apps.who.int/iris/bitstream/handle/10665/128703/e96854.pdf. Accessed 28 Aug 2023
WHO (2013b) People-centred health care: a policy framework. Available https://www.who.int/publications/i/item/9789290613176. Accessed 28 Aug 2023
WHO (2016a) Health literacy. Available https://www.who.int/healthpromotion/health-literacy/en/. Accessed 28 Aug 2023
WHO (2016b) Patient engagement: technical series on safer primary care. Available https://apps.who.int/iris/bitstream/handle/10665/252269/9789241511629-eng.pdf. Accessed 28 Aug 2023
WHO (2017) Shanghai declaration on promoting health in the 2030 Agenda for Sustainable Development. Available https://www.who.int/publications/i/item/WHO-NMH-PND-17.5 Accessed 28 Aug 2023
WHO (2023) Health promotion – health literacy. Available https://www.who.int/teams/health-promotion/enhanced-wellbeing/ninth-global-conference/health-literacy. Accessed 28 Aug 2023

Chapter 5
Supervision: A Tool for Good Health and Well-Being

Elise Kvalsund Bårdsgjerde, Bodil J. Landstad, Torstein Hole, Marit Kvangarsnes, and Berit Misund Dahl

Abstract This chapter presents supervision with the intention of strengthening good health and well-being. Supervision strategies for patients and service users and in groups amongst health professionals are described. Supervision aims to make individuals and organisations aware of the knowledge, experiences, and values underpinning their practice. This will enable them to become aware of their practical theory and increase the possibilities for change and development. Health-literate people and organisations are important for sustainable health services and in achieving Sustainable Development Goals (SDGs). Supervision is a tool for healthcare professionals to empower individuals and organisations for lifelong learning, as it

---

E. K. Bårdsgjerde (✉)
Department of Health Sciences in Ålesund, Norwegian University of Science and Technology (NTNU), Ålesund, Norway
e-mail: elise.k.bardsgjerde@ntnu.no

B. J. Landstad
Department of Health Sciences, Mid Sweden University, Östersund, Sweden

Unit of Research, Education and Development, Östersund Hospital, Östersund, Sweden

T. Hole
Medical Department, Ålesund Hospital, Møre og Romsdal Hospital Trust, Ålesund, Norway

Faculty of Medicine and Health Sciences, Norwegian University of Science and Technology (NTNU), Trondheim, Norway

M. Kvangarsnes
Department of Health Sciences in Ålesund, Norwegian University of Science and Technology (NTNU), Ålesund, Norway

Medical Department, Ålesund Hospital, Møre og Romsdal Hospital Trust, Ålesund, Norway

B. M. Dahl
Department of Health Sciences, Norwegian University of Science and Technology, Ålesund, Norway

Department of Public Health, University of Stavanger, Stavanger, Norway

T. Hole et al. (eds.), *Towards Sustainable Good Health and Well-being*,
https://doi.org/10.1007/978-3-031-61810-9_5

enables people's engagement in health promotion and treatment. Supervision is a valuable strategy for reaching the SDGs Good health and well-being (3) and Quality education (4).

Keywords Supervision · Pedagogical tools · Frame factors · Patient values · Organisational health literacy

5.1 Introduction

Health literacy is presented as a critical determinant of health and sustainable development in the future. Sustainability in health services requires autonomous and health-literate people who are able to assess, analyse, and comprehend health information in order to make decisions about their health (WHO 2017). There are great expectations in regard to increasing the level of the population's health literacy (Ministry of Health and Care Services 2019). These expectations place new demands on health professionals. Health professionals' communication, pedagogical competence, and professional knowledge are significant for supervision which is intended to increase health literacy (Ministry of Health and Care Services 2019).

A change in the roles and relationships between patient and health professionals have been described. The role of the patient has evolved from being a passive recipient of medical care to an active, empowered, and informed co-producer of health (WHO 2013a; Nylenna 2020). Increased patient participation through patient education, rehabilitation, supervision, and support has been emphasised as important for improving health literacy and shared decision-making. This change is in line with the underlying thinking of sustainable development. Health literacy empowers and drives equity in sustainable health development. Health-literate people have knowledge and skills to make the healthiest choices and decisions for themselves (WHO 2017). Supervision is based on the patient's preferences and experiences and facilitates a patient-centred approach. It is a strategy for strengthening health literacy and ensuring equal health services. Supervision may promote equitable quality education and facilitate lifelong learning in good health and well-being (SDG 3,4). An underlying thought in supervision is to stimulate the person's own thinking (Lauvås and Handal 2014). Continuous critical thinking linked to lifestyle choices is vital in developing good health and well-being.

Within public health, the role of the public health nurse has changed from acting as an expert to involving the parents as active participants at child health clinics (Dahl et al. 2014). Many problems cannot solely be solved by biomedical knowledge. This recognition served as the precursor to both health promotion strategies and the 1986 Ottawa Charter (WHO 1986; Dahl et al. 2014). Public health nursing is concerned with striking a balance between the role of experts and safeguarding service user involvement (Dahl 2016). One of the goals of supervision is to empower the service user so that they can make well-informed decisions for themselves and their families for good health and well-being (SDG 3).

Supervision is a tool which can be used for improving health literacy and creating health literate–friendly organisations. Examples from health-promoting, preventive, and therapeutic health services will be used to illustrate supervision in different contexts.

5.2 Supervision

Pedagogues, namely Gunnar Handal and Per Lauvås, have developed a pedagogical strategy, *the action and reflection model,* for vocational supervision that has been used in recent decades in professional educations and collegial supervision (Handal and Lauvås 1983, 1999; Lauvås et al. 2004; Lauvås and Handal 2014). This supervision strategy has been experienced as valuable in peer supervision in Higher Education (de Lange and Lauvås 2018).

We argue that the strategy is transferable to healthcare contexts to increase individual and organisational health literacy. The aim of the supervision strategy is that the person becomes aware of the knowledge, experience, and values on which the professional activity is based on rather than conveying the "right knowledge" (Bårdsgjerde et al. 2023). *The action and reflection model* is based on the person's own experiences and helps to draw connections between values and theoretical knowledge about thinking and acting in a specific situation (Lauvås and Handal 2014; Lauvås et al. 2016). It intends to make the person aware of own knowledge, experiences, and values, and Lauvås and Handal (2014) state that becoming aware of one's own knowledge increases the possibilities for change and development (Lauvås and Handal 2014).

An underlying thought in *the action and reflection model* is to empower the person to develop their knowledge base and stimulate critical thinking. Health literacy is a complex phenomenon related to the competencies of accessing, understanding, appraising, and applying health information in the domains of healthcare, disease prevention, and health promotion (Sørensen et al. 2012). Critical thinking is vital in this process, and we consider *the action and reflection model* to be valuable for strengthening health literacy. Health supervision presupposes that health professionals can use different forms of knowledge and pedagogical tools in their efforts to strengthen service users' critical thinking.

5.3 Pedagogical Tools

We will present tools from *the action and reflection model* (Lauvås and Handal 2014; Lauvås et al. 2016) that we consider to be valuable in supervision within a healthcare context (in Table 5.1). Based on practical challenges, the strategy stimulates the person to think about the underpinning assumptions of their practice.

Table 5.1 Pedagogical tools

Practical theory	Practical theory consists of values, experiences, and knowledge that underlie our actions. It is claimed that most people have little awareness of their own theory of practice (Handal and Lauvås 1999; Lauvås and Handal 2014). One goal of the supervision will be to help the person increase their understanding of their own practice theory. The prerequisite for change and development is that practice theory becomes available for analysis and critical appraisal (Handal and Lauvås 1999; Lauvås and Handal 2014). In a healthcare context, health professionals can be an important partner by asking open-ended questions related to the problem presented by the service user (Lauvås and Handal 2014; Bårdsgjerde et al. 2023)
Structure and progression	Structure and progression can help guide the conversation among its participants (Lauvås et al. 2016; de Lange et al. 2023). During conversations or consultations, health professionals often give advice immediately. In some situations, this may work well, because it solves a medical problem. However, giving advice too quickly may mean that health professionals do not have a complete understanding of the problem before giving such advice. To strengthen a person's health literacy, it is important to stimulate the person's critical thinking about different choices of action and their potential consequences (Bårdsgjerde et al. 2023)
Various perspectives	Often, issues are complex and can be analysed from different perspectives (Lauvås and Handal 2014). Exploring different perspectives may lead to a comprehensive understanding of the problem. Relevant perspectives in health supervision may be the patient, family, treatment, preventive, job, organisational, and the sustainability perspective. Different perspectives will emphasise different aspects of the problem field and might provide new insight (Bårdsgjerde et al. 2023)
Communication and metacommunication	Conversations consist of two levels: the content level and the relationship level (Lauvås and Handal 2014). In a healthcare context, it often becomes apparent that service users do not understand oral or written information. Using metacommunication, to talk about communication in supervision, may contribute to a mutual understanding and reciprocity between service user and healthcare professionals (Bårdsgjerde et al. 2023)

Transferred to a healthcare context, this may mean that the supervision strategy can help strengthen the service user's knowledge of their health challenges, as well as the consequences of various choices (Bårdsgjerde et al. 2023).

5.4 Individual Supervision

Individual supervision is a common form of knowledge sharing between patients and health professionals (Ministry of Health and Care Services 2019). Stressful life events, for example, being diagnosed with a chronic disease, can make individuals receptive to developing their knowledge and skills, often referred to as "teachable moments"(Rowlands et al. 2019). Research has shown that after a heart attack, the patient may be highly motivated to make lifestyle changes (Bårdsgjerde et al. 2019).

5.4.1 Relationships in Health Supervision

In health supervision, there often is an asymmetrical relationship, where health professionals possess expert knowledge. It will be important that health professionals base their work on the patient's understanding of the problem. Health professionals may learn from listening to patients' experiences (Bårdsgjerde et al. 2023). A study described patients' experience of breathlessness in COPD exacerbation, which is a dramatic situation and patients may experience the use of coercion during acute treatment (Kvangarsnes et al. 2013b). Loss of trust may be a consequence, and coping in acute situations is a relevant topic for supervision (Kvangarsnes et al. 2013a).

Health professionals should neither seek to instruct nor moralise, and health information must be adapted to the service user's circumstances and preferences. Many patients experience shame in their role as a patient, and this can be an obstacle to a positive learning process (Gulbrandsen 2006). The patient's feeling of shame is often underestimated, and health professionals should be aware of this phenomenon when working towards building health literacy.

In cases of supervision over time, it may be appropriate to ask the patient in advance to formulate what they wish to discuss. Listening to the patient's experience of the situation may give the patient's voice significance. By asking the patient open-ended questions, the patient may develop a better understanding of how they cope with the various challenges related to the situation (Bårdsgjerde et al. 2023).

5.4.2 Frame Factors and Structures

Time and access to health professionals are important in supervision. It might be useful if health professionals communicate the time available in each situation to the service user. This allows the service user to prioritise what is important to discuss. Many issues are complex, and it may be appropriate to have multiple consultations. Health professionals and service users should draw up a plan for the issues that need to be discussed (Bårdsgjerde et al. 2023). Research has emphasised time and continuity as important in follow-up of patients after a heart attack (Bårdsgjerde et al. 2022). Similar findings have been found in the palliative care setting. Continuity is important for patients and their next of kin so that they know who they should contact when the patient's condition worsens (Tarberg et al. 2022).

The importance of architecture and physical frames for consultation (Martinsen 2006) has been highlighted. In many institutions, patients do not have access to single rooms, and there is also a lack of rooms for private conversation. This makes it challenging to maintain confidentiality (Bårdsgjerde et al. 2023). A study found that the lack of facilities for private conversations hindered dialogue between physicians and patients in cardiac care (Bårdsgjerde et al. 2022). Rooms for consultations are often designed to fulfil several functions. An example is the doctor's office, which is planned for examinations, reporting, and supervision. This may make the patient feel that diagnostics take precedence, and that there is little room for personal conversations (Bårdsgjerde et al. 2023). Questions have been raised about what time, architecture, and knowledge do to the tone of space (Martinsen 2006; Kvangarsnes 2007). Standardised forms and checklists increasingly characterise consultations between healthcare professionals and patients. This may lead to less space for patients' stories and communication of their preferences. There is a risk that patients become an object rather than a participant in the process (Martinsen 2005). Health-literate patients mean active and engaged patients with confidence in their coping with the disease, decisions about lifestyle choices, and use of health services.

Increased standardisation in programmes and procedures has been found to challenge the use of professional judgement at child health centres (Dahl and Clancy 2015). Strategies to promote health are often designed to reach population groups, such as primary and secondary school classes (Dahl and Clancy 2015; Orkan 2019). Dahl and Clancy (2015) found that standardised education programmes implemented in school classes often revealed individual needs. Sometimes, public health nurses succeeded in applying standardised protocols to solve these individual needs: However, standardisation often hindered flexibility and the ability to make the correct clinical judgements.

5.4.3 Progression and Various Perspectives

Progression over time in supervision is important (Lauvås and Handal 2014; Lauvås et al. 2016). Health professionals should not proceed too quickly when providing advice. A common expectation is that the patient will present a problem, and the health professional will provide a solution (Bårdsgjerde et al. 2023). Shared decision-making is an example of how health professionals and patients can make joint decisions. Makoul and Clayman (2006) identified important elements of shared decision-making in encounters between physicians and patients. These elements have inspired the development of a tool for shared decision-making between patients and health professionals (Kienlin et al. 2020). The tool follows a structure: explaining the problem, presenting options and discuss pros and cons, identifying the patient values, preferences and discuss patient self-efficacy, health professionals provide their knowledge/recommendation, check and clarify understanding and make or defer decisions, and arrange further follow-up (Makoul and Clayman 2006). The process often takes place over time, and plans should be made.

In complex cases, follow-up consultations focusing on various perspective may be valuable. A common challenge in families with young children is problems with sleeping, and this may present challenges for the parents' professional life, social activity, and family life. The parents often need supervision over time to cope with the situation. The issues can be perceived as complex and unmanageable and needs to be explored from different perspectives. Relevant perspectives can be the child's, the sibling's, the parents', and the family's views. Clarifying the problem from different perspectives can help support parents in discovering new coping strategies (Bårdsgjerde et al. 2023).

5.4.4 *Communication and Metacommunication*

At the end of a supervision session, a summary of the conversation and decisions made should be carried out. Health professionals should ensure that the patient has understood the information provided and give the patient the opportunity to ask questions (Bårdsgjerde et al. 2023). One method for improving communication between patients and health professionals is called the "teach-back technique". The patient is asked to recall in their own words what the health professional has told them. The technique is often used to secure a common understanding between the patient and the health professionals (Talevski et al. 2020).

Health-literate organisations aim to make it easy for patients to navigate, understand, and use information and services to take care of their health (Brach et al. 2012; Brega et al. 2019). Written information prepared by health professionals is criticised for having a professional and bureaucratic language that is difficult for service users to understand (WHO 2013b; Hem and Nylenna 2021). Creating health literate–friendly organisations is one of the strategies to increase health literacy in populations globally. The Shanghai Declaration (WHO 2017) stated that health literacy was one of three pillars required to achieve SDG 3 ensuring healthy lives and promoting well-being for all people at all ages.

5.5 Supervision Among Colleagues

5.5.1 *Exercise in Peer Group Supervision*

In this section, we describe an exercise for peer group supervision among colleagues. The exercise has been applied in Higher Education (Lauvås et al. 2004, 2016; de Lange and Lauvås 2018; Kirkevold and De Lange 2023). We believe that this exercise is a valuable strategy to strengthen individual and organisational health literacy. Peer group supervision will be significant, for example, to analyse the degree to which organisations enable individuals to find, understand, and use information and services to inform health decisions and actions for themselves and others (Centers for Disease Control and Prevention (CDC) 2020). This is an important task for all health services. Organisational health literacy is complex, and highlighting various perspectives might be valuable. Examples of perspectives that might be relevant are the service user's e-health literacy, access to equipment, standardised equipment, cooperation between different levels in health services, legislation, clinical guidelines, and access to individual supervision.

Progression and structure are experienced as important in the exercise (de Lange and Lauvås 2018). The exercise provides practice in asking open-ended questions, which invite reflection and insight into the knowledge, experiences, and values underpinning their actions (Bårdsgjerde et al. 2023).

The exercise is suitable in professional communities with five to ten participants. The exercise is based on a specific problem as experienced by the professional. It should not be a general problem but rooted in a real situation related to strengthening organisational health literacy. This exercise consists of seven phases, as shown in Table 5.2. It takes approximately 90 minutes to complete, depending on the number of participants and the complexity of the chosen problem. The exercise has a

Table 5.2 The seven phases

1. Presentation	Each participant briefly presents a problem related to health literacy. It must be a real problem that you are facing and on which you want to shed light. It is important to maintain confidentiality
2. Choose a problem	The group chooses one of the presented problems to be elucidated further
3. Explanation of the problem	The person who presented the chosen problem provides supplementary information about the problem. The other participants cannot ask questions in this phase
4. Clarification of the problem and situation	By using the question and answers approach, you will now try to understand what the problem is about. Each participant poses in turn a simple question and the person receiving supervision answers. The session will continue until the situation/problem has been clarified. If you don't have any more questions, you can say "pass", and it is the next participant's turn
5. Own solutions	The person receiving supervision tells the group/health professional what s/he wants to do about the problem. The group leader notes the solution proposals formulated by the person on a large sheet of paper. The proposed solutions must be approved by the person receiving supervision
6. Advice	Each participant is given the opportunity to give one piece advice, and the session can take several rounds. At this time, neither the participants nor the person receiving supervision should comment or take a position on the advice given. The group leader notes the advice as formulated by the person who gave the advice on the sheet of proposed solutions
7. Evaluation of advice	The person receiving supervision now goes through the given advice. Relevant advice is marked with plus signs, while irrelevant advice is marked with minus signs. The person receiving supervision does not need to comment on the advice given. The other participants are unable to comment

Modified from Lauvås et al. (2016), de Lange and Lauvås (2018) Kirkevold and De Lange (2023)

leader who has a governing role. Lauvås et al. (2016) and de Lange and Lauvås (2018) recommend that the various phases must be followed as a procedure.

5.5.2 *Follow-Up: Reflections on Health Literacy and Sustainability*

- What learning outcomes were experienced by the person receiving supervision?
- How did the participants experience the tight structure in the exercise?
- How did the participants experience the use of open-ended questions?
- What pedagogical tools (practical theory, progression and structure, various perspectives, communication, and metacommunication) were applied?
- What learning outcomes did the participants experience?
- What can be transferred to individual or organisational supervision to strengthen health literacy and sustainability?
- How can supervision improve health literacy and sustainability?

It is important to be able to reflect on the experiences of the exercise to become aware of the importance of progression in supervision. By participating in the exercise, the participants will gain insight into and learn the value of using the various pedagogical tools in supervision and interaction with colleagues. This knowledge may be valuable and can be transferred to strengthen health literacy at an individual and organisational level.

5.6 Conclusion and Implications for Practice

We have presented experiences and theoretical perspectives about supervision to strengthen health literacy at both the individual and organisational levels. Health-literate people and organisations are important for sustainable health services and in achieving SDG 3 Good health and well-being. One of the goals of supervision is to make individuals and organisations aware of conditions for strengthening health literacy so that people can make good choices in order to achieve good health and well-being. There is a need for supervision at the individual and organisational levels to build health literacy and sustainable development. Supervision is a tool for healthcare professionals to empower individuals and organisations for lifelong learning. The requirements for health literacy will continue to change and require people to be able to adapt to new challenges in terms of climate and environment, economy, and social conditions.

We argue that there is a need to focus on supervision strategies to enhance individual and organisational health literacy in the future. Supervision can contribute to sustainable health services aiming to achieve good health and well-being through lifelong learning. Supervision for good health and well-being should be emphasised in curricula globally. Students in higher education within health care should be trained in supervision to strengthen health literacy at the individual and organisational levels.

References

Bårdsgjerde EK et al (2019) Patient's narratives of their patient participation in the myocardial infarction pathway. J Adv Nurs 75:1063–1073. https://doi.org/10.1111/jan.13931

Bårdsgjerde EK et al (2022) Physicians' perceptions of patient participation in the myocardial infarction pathway. Commun Med. https://doi.org/10.1558/cam.20555

Bårdsgjerde EK, Kvangarsnes M, Dahl BM (2023) Veiledning for å styrke helsekompetanse [Supervision for increasing health literacy]. In: Dahl BM, Bjørnsen HN (eds) Helsesykepleie i praksis [Public health nursing in practice]. Fagbokforlaget, Bergen

Brach C et al (2012) Ten attributes of health literate health care organizations. NAM Perspect. https://doi.org/10.31478/201206a

Brega AG et al (2019) Organizational health literacy: quality improvement measures with expert consensus. Health Lit Res Pract 3:e127–e146. https://doi.org/10.3928/24748307-20190503-01

Centers for Disease Control and Prevention (CDC) (2020) What is health literacy. Available https://www.cdc.gov/healthliteracy/learn/index.html. Accessed 28 Aug 2023

Dahl BM (2016) Helsesøstertjenesten i et innovasjonsperspektiv [The public nurse service in an innovation perspective]. In: Kvangarsnes M, Håvold JI, Helgesen Ø (eds) Innovasjon og entreprenørskap [Innovation and entrepreneurship] Fjordantologien 2015. Universitetsforlaget, Oslo

Dahl BM, Clancy A (2015) Meanings of knowledge and identity in public health nursing in a time of transition: interpretations of public health nurses' narratives. Scand J Caring Sci 29:679–687. https://doi.org/10.1111/scs.12196

Dahl BM, Andrews T, Clancy A (2014) Contradictory discourses of health promotion and disease prevention in the educational curriculum of Norwegian public health nursing: a critical discourse analysis. Scand J Public Health 42:32–37. https://doi.org/10.1177/1403494813502585

de Lange T, Lauvås P (2018) Kollegaveiledning i høyere utdanning – en empirisk analyse av veiledningssamtaler [Faculty peer mentoring in higher education – an analysis of peer conversations]. Uniped 41:259–274. https://doi.org/10.18261/issn.1893-8981-2018-03-07

de Lange T, Esterhazy R, Wittek L (2023) Peer group mentoring among faculty staff in higher education. In: De Lange T, Wittek L (eds) Faculty peer group mentoring in higher education – developing collegiality through organised supportive collaboration. Springer, Cham

Gulbrandsen P (2006) Skam i det medisinske rom [Shame in the medical room]. Gyldendal akademisk, Oslo

Handal G, Lauvås P (1983) På egne vilkår: en strategi for veiledning med lærere [On own terms: a strategy for mentoring with teachers]. Cappelen, Oslo

Handal G, Lauvås P (1999) På egne vilkår: en strategi for veiledning med lærere [On own terms: a strategy for mentoring with teachers], [Rev. utg.]. edn. Cappelen akademisk forl., Oslo

Hem E, Nylenna M (2021) Språk er også medisin [Language is also medicine]. Michael 18:7–13

Kienlin S, Eiring Ø, Kasper J (2020) Samvalg [Shared decision-making]. Michael 17:127–143

Kirkevold M, De Lange T (2023) Developing research supervision capacity in clinical health professions: structured peer group mentoring as collegial support in a research school context. In: De Lange T, Wittek L (eds) Faculty peer group mentoring in higher education – developing collegiality through organised supportive collaboration. Springer, Cham

Kvangarsnes M (2007) Helsearbeidaren som pedagog [The health worker as an educator]. In: Ekeland T-J, Heggen K (eds) Meistring og myndiggjering – reform eller retorikk? [Coping and empowerment – reform or rhetoric?]. Gyldendal Akademisk, Oslo

Kvangarsnes M et al (2013a) Intensive care unit nurses' perceptions of patient participation in the acute phase of chronic obstructive pulmonary disease exacerbation: an interview study. J Adv Nurs 69:425–434. https://doi.org/10.1111/j.1365-2648.2012.06021.x

Kvangarsnes M et al (2013b) Narratives of breathlessness in chronic obstructive pulmonary disease. J Clin Nurs 22:3062–3070. https://doi.org/10.1111/jocn.12033

Lauvås P, Handal G (2014) Veiledning og praktisk yrkesteori [Supervision and practical vocational theory], 3rd edn. Cappelen Damm akademisk, Oslo

Lauvås P, Lycke KH, Handal G (2004) Kollegaveiledning i skolen [Peer supervision in the school], 3. utg. edn. Cappelen akademisk forl., Oslo

Lauvås P et al. (2016) Kollegaveiledning med kritiske venner [Peer Supervosion with critical friends], 4. utg. edn. Cappelen Damm akademisk, Oslo

Makoul G, Clayman ML (2006) An integrative model of shared decision making in medical encounters. Patient Educ Couns 60:301–312. https://doi.org/10.1016/j.pec.2005.06.010

Martinsen K (2005) Samtalen, skjønnet og evidensen [Dialogue, judgement and evidence]. Akribe, Oslo

Martinsen K (2006) Care and vulnerability. Akribe, Oslo

Ministry of Health and Care Services (2019) Strategi for å øke helsekompetansen i befolkningen 2019–2023 [Strategy to increase health literacy in the population 2019–2023]. Available https://www.regjeringen.no/contentassets/97bb7d5c2dbf46be91c9df38a4c94183/strategi-helsekompetanse-uu.pdf. Accessed 28 Aug 2023

Nylenna M (2020) Fra lydighet til likeverd. Pasientmedvirkning i et historisk og helsepolitisk perspektiv [From obedience to equality. Patient participation in a historical and health policy perspective]. Michael 17:15–42

Orkan O (2019) From Saranac Lake to Shanghai: a brief history of health literacy. In: Orkan O et al (eds) International handbook of health literacy. Policy Press, Bristol

Rowlands G et al (2019) Health literacy and chronic conditions: a life course perspective. In: Orkan O et al (eds) International handbook of health literacy. Policy Press, Bristol

Sørensen K et al (2012) Health literacy and public health: a systematic review and integration of definitions and models. BMC Public Health 12:1–13. https://doi.org/10.1186/1471-2458-12-80

Talevski J et al (2020) Teach-back: a systematic review of implementation and impacts. PLoS One 15:e0231350. https://doi.org/10.1371/journal.pone.0231350

Tarberg AS et al (2022) Physicians' perceptions of patient participation and the involvement of family caregivers in the palliative care pathway. Health Expect 25:1945–1953. https://doi.org/10.1111/hex.13551

WHO (1986) Ottawa Charter for Health Promotion. Available https://www.euro.who.int/__data/assets/pdf_file/0004/129532/Ottawa_Charter.pdf. Accessed 4 Sept 2023

WHO (2013a) Exploring patient participation in reducing health-care-related safety risks. Available http://www.euro.who.int/__data/assets/pdf_file/0010/185779/e96814.pdf?ua=1. Accessed 4 Sept 2023

WHO (2013b) Health literacy The solid facts. Available https://apps.who.int/iris/bitstream/handle/10665/128703/e96854.pdf. Accessed 28 Aug 2023

WHO (2017) Shanghai declaration on promoting health in the 2030 Agenda for Sustainable Development. Available https://www.who.int/publications/i/item/WHO-NMH-PND-17.5. Accessed 28 Aug 2023

Chapter 6
Enhancing Health Literacy Through Sustainable Digital Healthcare Solutions: System Development and Usage Perspectives

Ainhoa Goienetxea, Anniken Karlsen, Anne Strand Alfredsen Larsen, Synnøve Opsahl Melseth, and Marie Flem Sørbø

Abstract This chapter summarises findings from an empirical study investigating how digital healthcare solutions should be developed to satisfy individual demands for understanding and managing healthcare information and activities. Despite the quick development of new digital healthcare services to accomplish service efficiency and cost-effectiveness, and at the same time supporting the achievement of a wide range of sustainable development goals, some users perceive challenges due to different age-related, physical, and cognitive starting points. The chapter offers a broad view of the development of digital healthcare solutions and considers literature and the perspectives of technologists, caregivers, and users through a qualitative approach using interviews and autoethnography. A main finding is that the development of digital healthcare solutions that enhance health literacy needs a comprehensive strategy, in which users, healthcare providers, family members, and other stakeholders should participate.

A. Goienetxea (✉)
Department of Intelligent Production Systems, School of Engineering Science, University of Skövde, Skövde, Sweden
e-mail: ainhoa.goienetxea@his.se

A. Karlsen
Department of ICT and Natural Sciences, Faculty of Information Technology and Electrical Engineering, Norwegian University of Science and Technology, Ålesund, Norway

A. S. A. Larsen
Department of Health Services Research, Ålesund Hospital, Møre and Romsdal Hospital Trust, Ålesund, Norway

S. O. Melseth
Department of Citizen Services, Ålesund Municipality, Ålesund, Norway

M. F. Sørbø
Department of Public Health and Nursing, Faculty of Medicine and Health Sciences, Norwegian University of Science and Technology, Trondheim, Norway

Competence Centre for Dental and Oral Health, Trondheim, Norway

T. Hole et al. (eds.), *Towards Sustainable Good Health and Well-being*,
https://doi.org/10.1007/978-3-031-61810-9_6

Keywords Digital healthcare solutions · User-centred design · Sustainability · Health literacy · Digital health literacy

6.1 Introduction

One of the main objectives of digital health can be perceived as generating a flow of patient data to devices and/or health professionals, in order to provide patients with information on their health and how to handle or improve it, for example, in large digital healthcare services, where the circulation of data is between clinicians, patients, and devices (Vayena et al. 2018). In Norway, *helsenorge.no* is an example of a digital healthcare solution (DHCS), whereby users get messages and letters from different health services, can book or keep track of appointments with general practitioners, and see the status of referrals to hospitals or specialist doctors, health centres, and municipal healthcare services. It is also possible to find a consolidated list of prescriptions for medicines and other items. Whilst a motive for offering *helsenorge.no* and other services is to provide what the Norwegian Directorate of Health describes as quality-assured information and self-service solutions (Helsedirektoratet 2020), within the complexity that exists in the current organisation of health services, one cannot ignore the fact that a significant part of the population lack the necessary skills to use and benefit from digital tools for promoting health and delivering healthcare. In other words, there is a deficiency in (digital) health literacy. As far back as 2006, Norman and Skinner (2006) warned that half of the adult population in the United States and Canada lacked the skills necessary to effectively engage in an information-rich society and that DHCSs provide little value for such citizens. Whilst the population's digital skills and digital use have increased since 2006, findings show that, amongst others, people aged 60 and over still experience challenges with digital participation (Bjønness et al. 2021). At the same time, such people constitute a group with an increasing demand for general practitioner (GP) health consultations in Norway (Statistics Norway 2022a). In 2030, for the first time in Norwegian history, the number of those aged 65 and over will be higher than the number of younger people (aged 0 to 19) according to Statistics Norway (2020). Furthermore, one out of five of the whole population will be over 70 years old by 2060. We can therefore see a significant increase in ageing in Norway for many years to come. This constitutes a double challenge, the demographic development (more elderly people), and the fact that DHCSs are needed to cope with the increase in demand for healthcare. If DHCSs realise their potential for improving citizens' health and thus contribute as a useful tool for developing sustainable health services, the gap between what is provided, and what people can access, should be recognised and remedied (Norman and Skinner 2006). Regarding the latter, and knowing that several people struggle with the use of technology, the overarching question raised and addressed in this chapter is:

How should sustainable digital healthcare solutions be developed to enhance health literacy whilst adapting to various users' needs?

The aim in this chapter is, therefore, to investigate what is required of health services, what is required of the users and potentially their relatives, and not least, what is required of technologists and others developing the DHCSs.

6.2 Theoretical Background

Motivators for the continuous development of digital healthcare services can be found in concrete digital health vision statements by the World Health Organization (WHO). WHO recognises that digitalisation has the potential to radically change health outcomes if adequate resources are allocated to governance, people, and processes. Sufficient resources are needed to provide opportunities for necessary adaptions to increasingly digitised health systems and services. Together with national strategies and visions for healthcare digitalisation, digital health can improve both the efficiency and cost-effectiveness of care (WHO 2021).

Contemporary DHCSs are developed to provide improved access to health-related information to care providers (Shaw et al. 2018) as well as to facilitate patient engagement (Birnbaum et al. 2015). The aim is to make it easier for the public to actively participate as patients in a complex healthcare system (Shaw et al. 2018), and to make it more effective for healthcare workers experiencing an increased workload due to the increment in the number of elderly patients in need of care (Shah et al. 2021). This calls for an additional need for skills complementary to health literacy, so-called digital health literacy, i.e. the ability to appraise health information from electronic sources and apply the knowledge gained for addressing or solving a health-related problem (Smith and Magnani 2019), which is also seen as an extension of health literacy (Palumbo et al. 2022; Dunn and Hazzard 2019). Necessary skills associated with the latter are, among others, the ability to use computers and applications such as search engines to accomplish tasks efficiently (Norman and Skinner 2006; Smith and Magnani 2019). Digital health literacy is further perceived as a crucial factor for cost reduction in healthcare and for limiting the sector's environmental impact; thus, it plays a fundamental role in achieving sustainable healthcare services (Palumbo et al. 2022). Additionally, Dunn and Hazzard (2019) state that technological solutions can either advance health literacy or be a barrier and that in order to be effective, solutions should go beyond simply building literacy and numeracy skills, to building functional and critical skills. Santana et al. (2021) emphasise that in recent literature, health literacy is related to individual capabilities and to an organisation's ability to make information regarding health and health services equitably accessible and comprehensible. Thus, an expanded definition can increase awareness of the role that various organisations play in ensuring that individuals can access, understand, and act on the health information and services they provide. Also, a broader definition may help support efforts to integrate health literacy principles into policy (Santana et al. 2021).

Furthermore, the development of DHCSs support the achievement of various Sustainable Development Goals (SDGs) included in the 2030 Agenda for Sustainable Development (United Nations 2015). Regarding, for example, the impact of DHCSs on SDG 3, i.e. to "Ensure healthy lives and promote well-being for all at all ages", it is, according to Gerlach (2019), obvious. The opportunity to access healthcare services wherever the patient is and be able to provide universal health coverage is enormously increased using DHCSs. Even language or cultural barriers could be overcome using DHCSs. Gerlach (2019) also finds connections between SDGs 5, 10, 12, and 13 and DHCSs. As regards SDG 5, to "Achieve gender equality and empower all women and girls", Gerlach (2019) points to applications enabling women to track their menstrual cycle or general health, which provide the potential to empower women to prevent pregnancies, or to prepare and plan for conceiving a child or ensure a healthy pregnancy. Regarding SDG 10, to "Reduce inequality within and among countries", Gerlach (2019) emphasises that millions of people struggle to access basic healthcare services in developing countries. In such situations artificial intelligence (AI) based expert systems can, among others, provide high-level competence and as such contribute to the democratisation of medical knowledge and information. Important to note though is that such solutions need high-quality data sets and security standards regarding data privacy and protection (Gerlach 2019).

When it comes to SDG 12, to "Ensure sustainable consumption and production patterns", Gerlach (2019) emphasises that, for example, substituting paper-based patient records with digital copies leads to a major reduction in CO_2 emissions. The same goes for replacing physical visits with telemedicine. It is, of course, also important to consider the costs that come with DHCSs, for example, the requirements of devices and infrastructure that consume energy and produce electronic waste. Finally, when it comes to SDG 13, to "Take urgent action to combat climate change and its impacts", Gerlach (2019) highlights the use of DHCSs to promote behavioural changes by, e.g. facilitating a healthier diet for healthier living, correlated with more environmentally friendly lifestyles. In addition, AI-based expert systems, solutions making use of emerging technologies like social robots, virtual reality, and augmented reality technologies have caught practitioners' and researchers' interest within the digital health area. For example, immersive virtual reality–based exercise video games are increasingly being used as a supportive intervention in rehabilitation programmes to promote engagement in physical activity (Shah et al. 2022a, b).

Besides the many opportunities and benefits seen in developing DHCSs, some challenges to their use also exist. Heponiemi et al. (2022) show that people over the age of 60 are associated with a lower likelihood of using online services for receiving test results, renewing medical prescriptions, and scheduling appointments. Heponiemi et al. (2022) also found that good or average digital competence counters this age-related decline in online service use until the age of 80. After that age, good digital competence does not contribute to maintaining high usage levels.

These findings implicate that means should be implemented to prevent these older members of society from being digitally excluded. One way to increase online service use is to offer older people user support and another may be to focus on hedonic motivation associated with using the services (Heponiemi et al. 2022). However, challenges associated with the use of DHCSs are not just limited to the age of the user and this should not come as a surprise. More than 20 years ago, Nielsen (1999) was already pointing out potential difficulties *in designing Web usability.* For example, individuals with impaired vision may have difficulties using software with small text or buttons, or software that does not have proper accessibility features such as text-to-speech or sharp contrast modes. Persons with mobility impairments may have difficulties using a mouse or keyboard or may require the use of assistive technologies such as speech recognition software or on-screen keyboards. Individuals with cognitive impairments may have difficulties with tasks that require sustained attention or the processing of substantial amounts of information. Individuals who have hearing impairments may have difficulties using software that relies heavily on audio output. Also, physical and cognitive abilities are usually reduced as people age in a way that affects their ability to use software. To address these and other challenges related to diversities in people's states of health when facing technological products and services, a variety of universal design recommendations and regulations have been formulated. For example, the European Union's (2016) (EU) Web Accessibility Directive (WAD) aims at making public sector websites and mobile applications more accessible, harmonising varying standards within the EU, and reducing barriers for developers of accessibility-related products and services. The same applies to the Web Content Accessibility Guidelines 2.1 (WCAG) standard which became operative on 1 February 2023. According to the World Wide Web Consortium, the WCAG 2.1 standard (2018) is based on four design principles:

1. Perceivable: making sure users can recognise and use a service with the senses that are available to them.
2. Operable: making sure users can find and use the content, regardless of how they choose to access it.
3. Understandable: making sure people can understand the content and how the service works.
4. Robust: making sure the content can be interpreted reliably by a wide variety of user agents

The design principles are supported by 13 guidelines, and each of these is further broken down into specific success criteria or requirements that the service should meet. As regards accessibility, it should be noted that the Web accessibility initiative (WAI) emphasises that accessibility is closely related to usability and inclusion, in creating a Web that works for everyone, whereby accessibility addresses discrimination aspects related to equivalent user experience for people with disabilities, usability is about designing products to be efficient, effective, and satisfying, whilst inclusion is about diversity and the involvement of everyone to the greatest extent possible (WAI 2016).

Whilst WAD focuses on software-related aspects associated with information systems development, the WHO (2021) focuses on strategic aspects emphasising that digital health should be an integral part of health priorities and that countries require institutional support for the development and consolidation of national e-health and/or digital health strategies and the implementation of action plans. However, a major concern regarding DHCSs is security aspects and ethical issues, a theme addressed in the review by Vayena et al. (2018) where the focus is on ethical and policy challenges of innovation in digital health. The authors highlight different requisites to be fulfilled for digital health applications to have a tangible effect on public and individual health. Access to data is seen as vital for the development of innovative diagnostic, therapeutic, and monitoring tools. In addition to this, digital health products are required to comply with countries' privacy, data protection, and data security requirements. Vayena et al. (2018) also state that robust and transparent accountability mechanisms should ensure the precise identification of responsibility for use of data and their consequences on individuals, families, and communities and that evidence of safety and efficacy is crucial for the success of digital health in fostering trust in both developers and regulators which will, in turn, facilitate the uptake of digital health by healthcare providers and lead to a fair sharing of benefits of digital health innovation.

6.3 Methodology

This study combines insights from scientific literature and empirical information from interviews with users and gathers the views of researchers with diverse backgrounds and experiences with the development and use of DHCSs. By combining these insights, the aim is to contribute to a more comprehensive understanding of crucial factors that should be kept in mind when creating DHCSs that enhance health literacy and cater to individuals with diverse physical and cognitive backgrounds rather than limiting the investigation to just one or two information sources. Thus, this study rests on different approaches for shedding light on the research topic, which relates to methodological triangulation, which, per se, is important for validation and hence strengthens the study's trustworthiness (Saunders et al. 2019).

6.3.1 Interviews with Users

Interviews were conducted in Norway with people aged 67 and above, as it is considered that this group of people struggles the most with digital participation (Bjønness et al. 2021). The participants' perspectives on the digitalisation of society and their thoughts on using DHCSs regarding aspects like user-friendliness and accessibility were given particular attention.

6.3.1.1 Data Collection

Since the main aim was to obtain nuanced insights into users' perceptions of DHCSs and not to quantify, we used semi-structured interviews with open-ended questions to collect data from the user's perspective (Kvale and Brinkmann 2015). Open-ended questions were included as they provide the desired flexibility and ability to adapt to the current situation (Saunders et al. 2019). Additionally, open-ended questions allow informants to speak freely and provide them with an opportunity to emphasise their feedback when they have thorough insights or strong meanings or experiences to share (Tjora 2012). Semi-structured interviews also allow for digressions so that topics can be explored from perspectives not considered by the interviewer in advance (ibid.).

Seven participants were recruited from a municipal course initiative called "The Digital Senior". Thus, the informants were purposively sampled aiming for exploration and illustrations of the topic under study (Saunders et al. 2019). The interviews were conducted in connection with these meetings, with informants who volunteered to participate. Three interviews were conducted in total in January and February 2023. The interviews were performed by one researcher taking notes and lasted for 15–30 minutes. One interview was conducted with two informants together (two females), another one was conducted with one individual informant (male), and the last interview was conducted with four informants (three females, one male). Before the interviews, an interview guide was made based on the study's purpose of shedding light on the user perspective in DHCSs. The interview guide was developed by one researcher and discussed and agreed upon among all five researchers.

6.3.1.2 Data Analysis

The interviews were analysed by following Creswell's (2014) procedure for data analysis and interpretation. To prepare and organise the data for analysis, the researchers read the interview notes to get an overview and holistic impression of the data (Kvale and Brinkmann 2015). One researcher coded the data using paper, pencil, and a Word processor and established relevant categories. The initial coding process identified preliminary codes, which were processed through seven categories and finalised into two main themes. The initial codes, categories, and final themes were discussed among the researchers. The resulting themes and selected citations are presented in the result section.

6.3.2 One's Own Experiences and Views

The mapping of one's own experience and views as a source of insight into the subject matter is inspired by autoethnography, which is commonly used in sociology, anthropology, and cultural studies and is a way of understanding and interpreting the world through a personal, subjective lens. More specifically, autoethnography can be described as a qualitative research method that values researchers' individual experiences for describing and critiquing cultural beliefs, practices, and experiences (Adams et al. 2015). The approach followed in this study leans towards what Anderson (2006) refers to as analytical autoethnography, i.e. an attempt to establish connections between the researchers' experiences and the wider context through documentation. The subjective understanding and experiences can be broadly considered as cultural expressions and thus help to challenge and develop the understanding of knowledge (Klevan et al. 2019).

The mapping of these 'self-experiences' and views was carried out by a team of five researchers, including two technologists and three caregivers. The caregivers have long-term experience working with DHCSs in hospitals and primary care in Norway. A reflection has been made based on these experiences with a twofold perspective: what the caregivers experienced by using DHCSs themselves to support and have diverse communication with patients as well as the feedback they got from patients and family members after using DHCSs. The technologists have a background in informatics and health informatics and have comprehensive experience in the development and implementation of diverse DHCSs. The work started by reflecting, talking, and exchanging personal experiences related to DHCSs, highlighting challenges, and gaining insight into each other's perspectives. Furthermore, scientific literature on international and national guidelines related to the digitalisation of healthcare services and related regulations was analysed. The connection between DHCSs as part of the development of sustainable health services and the topic of health literacy was also a natural part of these reflections. The results of our conversations are formulated in two texts that describe the perspectives of the technologists and caregivers. The views of the researchers (the two texts) are summarised in the *Results* section and are mainly based on the extended professional experience (20–25 years) in researching the implementation and use of DHCSs (technologists) and the extended professional experience (20–30 years) in offering healthcare services (caregivers). The researchers' experience is based on their professional background working in Norway, Sweden, and Spain.

6.4 Results

Results from the interviews with the users and the researchers' perspectives are presented in this section.

6.4.1 Interviews with Users

6.4.1.1 Competence and Need for Training

Competence was a prominent topic in the interviews. The informants highlighted both the need for competence and the need for having the ability to gain needed competence. Several informants said that their current knowledge was achieved on their own initiative and that they were self-taught and had not received any training. The informants further emphasised the importance of being brave and confident enough to try out the digital solutions themselves and not being afraid of making mistakes. The informants expressed that few opportunities to attend courses or other educational and training activities where they can go for help exist, which is illustrated in the following citation:

> No one has got any kind of training in how to use digital healthcare solutions, and we miss the opportunity for education.

Some informants pointed out the need to lean on a third party to cope with DHCSs. Receiving help from a third party was described as much appreciated; however, the informants also emphasised that this is not an option for all people their age. In practice, this means that they have nowhere to turn for help. Another highlighted aspect was that receiving help from a third party not always was carried out sustainably, as the following citation illustrates:

> We ask our grandchildren for help, and they just do their thing...So we do not know how to do this ourselves the next time or we forget how to...

The informants therefore pointed to the need for courses or venues for training and guidance and opportunities for meeting others for discussions and exchanging experiences, which are seen as important and contribute to further interest and curiosity in using DHCSs. The informants pointed out that some courses or initiatives to help seniors become more digitally skilled do exist and that these are useful. However, information about these events is often digital, and finding and attending these initiatives happen mainly on an individual basis.

6.4.1.2 Freedom of Choice: Opportunities for Personalisation

Another issue brought up by the informants was that the users are different and have diverse needs and expectations regarding DHCSs. The informants said that many seniors are digitally aware and want to cope with digital services, but also emphasised that not all seniors want to "go digital" and thus prefer information like they have been used to, for example, by letters. The informants discussed potential reasons for this, and as one of the informants said:

> Of course many have gone digital, but there are some that are stubborn and stuck-in-the-mud persons, pardon my language.

In this context, the informants also emphasised that alternatives to DHCSs are valuable and stressed that no one should be forced into using DHCSs. They highlighted the need for diversification that it should be possible to opt out of digital solutions and that alternative solutions for those preferring not to go digital should exist. The informants said that it is still nice to talk to human beings sometimes, by, for example, having the opportunity to call the bank or the doctor's office.

Even if the informants did point out challenges with DHCSs, they also reflected upon the current situation as satisfactory. They pointed out solutions they found useful and expressed that they were able to find good information online. However, they did stress that it is important to be aware of the possible vulnerable context surrounding health issues. The informants pointed out that experiencing challenges with DHCSs may become an additional burden in an already vulnerable situation. A vulnerable situation where something might be wrong with your health or well-being might make it more difficult to cope with digital healthcare applications or even to get hold of all the information that is needed.

6.4.1.3 User-Friendliness

Regarding the user-friendliness of DHCSs, the informants pointed to two levels: the system level and the personal/single-user level. At the system level, the informants expressed some frustrations regarding the multitude of different digital solutions they had to deal with. Different healthcare providers, such as public or private hospitals or general practitioners, use different solutions to communicate with their patients. Thus, the informants described it as challenging to know where to find information, e.g. scheduled appointments or results from examinations or other encounters with different healthcare providers. This is illustrated in the following citation:

> There are quite a few systems you must deal with…What goes where? [...] And the hospital communicates both digitally and by letters…and I think we get text messages as well.

Thus, the experience of the use of DHCSs can be seen as overwhelming for the users, as illustrated by the blunt response from one informant on the question regarding the need for DHCSs: "No more data!"

Logging in to different digital applications was perceived as time-consuming both due to occasional unfamiliarity with the technology and due to what was perceived as slow systems. Additionally, system errors and system changes were also mentioned as a source of frustration due to a feeling of having to "do or learn everything over again". Also, the user-friendliness of healthcare applications' user interfaces was pointed out as an issue, since the seniors may have vision impairment, or their hands may be shaking, making actual use a challenge.

Furthermore, the informants also described cumbersome and time-consuming login procedures due to data protection issues. Although they understood the need for high security and confidentiality levels, the informants questioned the levels being this high and further expressed that it sometimes seemed as if security issues were prioritised over maintaining user-friendliness.

At the personal/single-user level, some issues of user-friendliness were closely related to the level of competence, but the informants also emphasised that DHCSs should be intuitive enough for the users to manage by themselves. The informants pointed out the need for "knowing how to do it", e.g. zooming or enhancing font size:

> ...if you are supposed to adjust the font size on your device, you need to know how to do it. [...] You need to know how to adapt digital solutions to your own needs.

6.4.2 Researchers' Own Experiences

6.4.2.1 Technologists' Perspectives

Regarding the wide range of DHCSs available, including patient portals, mobile health apps, telemedicine systems, and a variety of wearable technology, various systems are created with general users in mind, whilst others are created specifically for those facing unique difficulties brought on by diseases and associated widespread health issues. Due to such differences in user groups and demands, several issues, such as usability and user training, should be considered when developing DHCSs. Correspondingly, rules and guidelines are developed to help ensure accessibility, and several design issues should be considered and addressed as part of DHCS development.

For a long time, the term "*universal design*" has been considered a desirable objective. However, liminal cases may be forgotten, i.e. single individuals who do not fit into the general picture of the users. The effect of a specific disease can vary not only from person to person but also throughout the course of the disease. These issues should also be considered, and alternative service offerings should be provided, so that people are not excluded when, for example, their health condition has changed so that current digital health offerings are no longer accessible or useful. In addition, besides addressing accessibility and interrelated issues like usability and inclusion, whilst developing DHCSs, other technical issues also should be handled, such as *interoperability*, *reliability*, *security*, and *privacy* issues. As regards *interoperability*, it is vital to consider how DHCSs can integrate with other systems and platforms to provide a seamless user experience. As regards personal health information and its *security*, it is evident that it should be protected from unauthorised access. This may involve implementing strong encryption and authentication measures, whilst from a health legislative perspective, this issue complies with various regulations and laws. Also, as regards *reliability* from a medical perspective, it is vital to ensure that the service is reliable and available when users need it. In worst-case scenarios, the consequences of missing health information might be fatal for some users. *Reliability*, as seen from a technical viewpoint, may involve implementing robust failover and disaster recovery systems, whilst from a health perspective, this is seen to demand precise information registered by health professionals in the

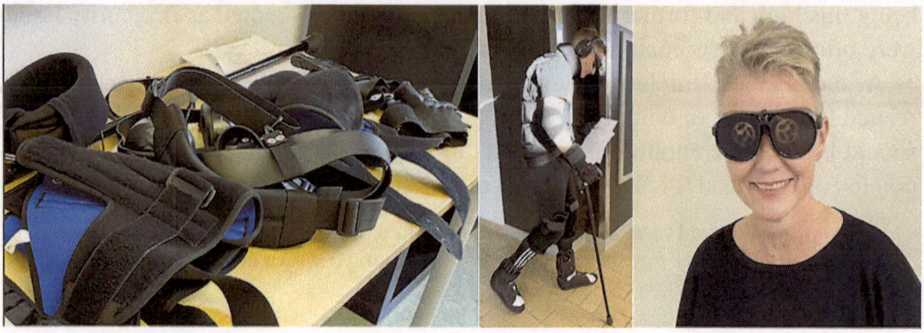

Fig. 6.1 Age simulation suit components. One of the authors wearing glasses simulating an eye disorder. (Photo: author's own)

first place. In any case, healthcare services, whether based on human-to-human interaction or based on human-computer interaction or a mix of the two, need to focus on a form of communication and health content adapted to the individual's needs. Otherwise, there is a risk of DHCSs ending up as generic, sterile interaction services that suit "most people" but not individuals with all their unique functional and mental requirements and specific health challenges. This was a point on which the authors focused particularly after using an age simulation suit in a class of nursing students. While wearing the suit, the nursing students were mostly thinking about general health concerns and the corresponding care needs of elderly people. However, the authors, as researchers, also focused on the suit's potential within the context of information systems development, particularly as a revelation for systems developers aiming at user-centred designs for people with various disabilities. See Fig. 6.1.

6.4.2.2 Caregivers' Perspectives

It is easy to highlight both the advantages and potential challenges of DHCSs. For example, there is a concern that because of the large variety of users and user needs, there is a risk of creating systems that digitally exclude those needing health services the most, such as the elderly and those with disabilities who find it challenging to benefit from using DHCSs.

On the positive side, contemporary technology brings a lot of advantages. From a therapeutic and clinical standpoint, maintaining relationships with loved ones is essential for good health and is made possible by a variety of technological options. People with special needs or those in nursing homes can communicate by utilising a tablet or computer to converse and see their partners, kids, grandchildren, or friends. Sometimes patients can manage to organise the meetings themselves, whilst others need a little support from the staff. Being in touch with loved ones more frequently might be beneficial in preventing loneliness and despair. Additionally, it is becoming more usual for patients to have consultations online, avoiding the need to travel to physically attend a doctor's appointment.

Another example of the use and impact of technology on health is the use of global positioning systems (GPS), which are used more frequently by people with cognitive disabilities. Those who are staying with their family can use GPS to leave the house by themselves while their family monitor their whereabouts. As a result, people with dementia, as well as their families, will gain more independence. This also makes it possible for patients to exercise more, which in turn improves their overall health – both physical and mental – as well as their quality of life.

Another viewpoint to consider is how people seeking care use DHCSs. To provide care services and DHCSs, healthcare service providers also need to modify their organisations and processes. For instance, it should be regularly assessed whether the DHCSs provided to patients are appropriate as their cognitive or physical capacities decline. Services provided through various channels should also be coordinated so that the patient's quality of treatment is independent of the service they select. The authors also contend that providing high-quality care should always take precedence over profit-driven decisions. Finally, the authors recognise the requirement that, before deployment, a clear strategy for maximising the benefits of using DHCSs and integrating them into the current working standards should be devised. A frequent problem is the medical staff's inability to use the newly specified DHCSs due to a lack of preparedness or expertise. Medical staff who are already overworked could feel unappreciated, unmotivated, and stressed because of this. Therefore, it is essential to make sure that the required conditions are met before introducing fresh strategies for dealing with DHCSs. Furthermore, the authors see it as essential that medical experts' advice should be taken into consideration when developing DHCSs.

6.5 Discussion

The aim of this study was to investigate how sustainable digital healthcare solutions should be developed to enhance health literacy while adapting to various users' needs. The data material has provided a more holistic understanding of the user needs that must be taken into account in order to develop sustainable DHCS that strengthen users' health literacy. Our informants emphasised that DHCSs must be user-friendly at both an individual level and a system level. This means that the DHCSs must be as intuitive as possible and adapted to age-related cognitive and physical challenges. At the system level, there should be more standardised approaches to DHCSs, for example, in terms of user interfaces and login procedures. The latter also points to the need for organisational health competence, which affects the user indirectly and is an important part of creating sustainable health services. To become more self-reliant and health literate, the informants also pointed out the importance of the opportunity to increase their own expertise and to exercise, preferably together with like-minded people. Such meeting points or arenas for training should be publicly available and be a low-threshold service where you can *come as you are*. The informants were also concerned that DHCSs should offer the possibility for customisation to meet different individual needs, expectations, and challenges. Customisation on such a scale ranges from those who may just need a little "nudge" to become independent to those who do not want to use digital solutions and should not be forced into using them but be able to receive what they need and communicate in other ways, such as by letter and telephone. The themes raised by the informants are important to consider for both DHCS developers and caregivers. The themes correspond well with our reflections and experiences as researchers in this area.

The importance of, and need for, digital competencies is one of the findings from the investigation as a crucial aspect to consider while creating DHCSs. This is an aspect both emphasised in literature and by the informants. Developing DHCSs that exclude large user groups due to demanding requirements as regards digital skills may be considered discriminating and an aspect that may go against various SDGs. While active, participatory, and responsible individuals are described as the ideal that policies and services should be oriented towards (Askheim and Andersen 2023), there may be some concerns about how useful such an ideal is when some of the largest user groups in healthcare probably do not fulfil it. Important to note regarding this aspect is that whilst health literacy encompasses both a personal and organisational perspective, the latest definitions of the term emphasise people's ability to use information rather than just understand it (personal perspective) at the same time acknowledging that responsibilities also exist at an organisational level to enable health literacy (Helsedirektoratet 2020). Several considerations, as stated by law and emphasised via various best design practices, should be considered carefully when designing DHCSs to ease the burden on individual users. An especially important aspect to keep in mind is the many demands commonly put on individuals regarding skills of general literacy, critical thinking, numeracy, comprehension, and the ability to seek information to participate in understanding and managing healthcare as emphasised by Smith and Magnani (2019) and supported by both interview statements and the authors' own experiences. Addressing these demands puts a huge responsibility on systems engineers, and public and private organisations, and is both complex and complicated. Generally, building information systems meeting the needs and preferences of diverse users is a challenging task requiring a combination of careful planning, user research, and flexibility both in design and in information systems implementation. A few approaches to consider may be to start identifying user needs and preferences. This can be done through interviews, surveys, focus groups, and usability testing. Customisation of DHCSs can be achieved, for instance, by offering various navigation and display options based on the roles or preferences of users, i.e. by adhering to WCAG 2.1 (2018) and other well-known principles for functional design. Also, since different users may find it difficult to access the information system itself, it is advisable to offer a variety of access methods, such as mobile access in addition to Web-based access and access through desktop programmes. Along with considering probable functional and cognitive limitations among those expected to utilise the DHCSs, it is critical to consider the likelihood that certain users may lack broader knowledge about digital solutions. This raises the notion that providing proper training and support for users of the system in the form of documentation, tutorials, and in-person training sessions may be the most crucial strategy and the one that is frequently overlooked while providing DHCSs. This can help users become proficient in system usage, and at the same time, system designers can gain valuable insight into how the services offered may be improved. This is in line with the results from the interviews and with the challenges presented in the literature. More competence and arenas for learning and training are important for improving health literacy, which further contributes to more sustainable health services. Meeting places where one can discuss relevant topics on how to handle digitalisation are also important. Such meeting places enable users to share experiences and may serve as an arena for jointly solving problems or discussing issues connected to digital solutions. Furthermore, such meetings provide opportunities for training and familiarisation with digital solutions. Such meeting places could also serve as a source for feedback from users to developers or system owners. For DHCSs to be of value, people need training in how to best use/navigate them. This is true for both caregivers who use the DHCSs to communicate with patients and others, and for caretakers themselves who are expected to utilise the services offered. Furthermore, user-friendliness should be considered both on a system level and an individual level. Developers should engage the end user in designing and developing DHCSs to tailor the user interfaces and make applications suited to the users' actual needs. Systems should be designed and developed in such a way that users intuitively understand them, thus strengthening both organisational and individual health literacy (Helsedirektoratet 2020).

6.6 Ethical Considerations

The informants were recruited on a voluntary basis in connection with "the digital senior" courses. One of the researchers provided an orientation about this study, and course attendants volunteered to participate and thus gave their informed consent to be interviewed either alone or in groups. Informed consent is essential according to, for example, the Helsinki Declaration (Førde 2014; Halvorsen and Jerpseth 2016). In the representation of findings from the interviews, both descriptively and through citations, informants are anonymised and cannot be recognised. This study is not covered by the Health Research Act and is, therefore, not subject to approval by the Regional Committees for Medical and Health Research Ethics (REK).

This study has also collected data through an autoethnographic approach by drawing on the researchers' knowledge of DHCS from different perspectives (technologists and caregivers). Thus, the researchers' proximity to the topic, and not objectivity, becomes both an epistemological starting point and point of arrival

(Conquergood 2002). Ellis et al. (2011) point out that researchers do not exist in isolation, i.e. those around them will be implicated in the research process. It is particularly important to be aware of this when conducting autoethnographic studies since relational considerations must be regarded as a crucial dimension in this type of research. The researcher must therefore, in addition to the methodological approach and literature, consider how others may experience the topic under study and use personal experiences to describe it and make relevant characteristics known to both insiders and outsiders (Ellis et al. 2011). The conclusions presented in this chapter are thus not an objective truth but descriptions of the researchers' own experiences and reflections as they appear to us as the authors of this chapter.

6.7 Limitations

The chosen methodology to conduct the research may have some limitations which are detailed in the paragraphs below.

Not using audio or video recordings may reduce the accuracy and constitute a risk for researcher bias. On the other hand, recording interviews may make informants more cautious and sceptical to share information (Saunders et al. 2019). We have explained the reason for interviewing seniors in this study. However, there is always a possibility for including more informants both from the senior population and from other groups, such as people with various kinds of cognitive and physical disorders or even developers. This is certainly an interesting avenue for further research. Additionally, the results of interviews reflect the private opinions and experiences of the informants.

Autoethnography is a method employed to consider and comprehend one's own reflections and experiences as well as how these interact with the world. In this study, the opinion of five researchers with diverse backgrounds was considered. While writing this chapter, their different experiences have been discussed, and feedback from the rest of the authors has been included. The inclusion of more researchers (both technologists and caregivers) could identify additional important insights not reflected in this chapter. The researchers have experience from mainly working in Nordic countries; experience from working in other parts of the world may raise other types of concerns or challenges not identified in this chapter.

This chapter has focused mainly on groups with different ages, physical, and cognitive starting points. However, other groups should also be considered such as poorly integrated immigrants, especially women immigrants, or whom apart from a lack of digital health literacy, language may be an additional barrier (Statistics Norway 2022b). Young people with a lack of bureaucratic competence on rights and obligations may also have a higher probability of digital exclusion (Statistics Norway 2022b).

6.8 Conclusions

This chapter provides a broad perspective on how to develop sustainable DHCSs considering user perspectives, caregiver perspectives, and technologist perspectives to enhance health literacy. The analysis of scientific literature, interviews with users, and mapping of individual experiences of the researchers have been used to conduct the study. The main findings of this chapter include the need for taking a broader perspective when developing DHCSs considering not just the general population and their needs but also the needs of individuals and caregivers.

From a global health perspective, WHO (2023) has stated that all too often, products are developed with the unfortunate approach that "if you build it, they will use it". However, this is far from being true: it is necessary to take a proactive, systematic approach for developing innovations based on user needs. DHCSs open new opportunities for providing healthcare. Furthermore, with the pace of technological change, the use of DHCSs will only increase in the future to support healthcare providers to offer more accessible and better care. Building systems for users with varying needs and preferences motivates the conduction of user research and testing to understand how people use the service and to identify areas for system improvements. General principles for useful design are just part of the answer. It is important to have deep knowledge of how various disabilities affect what is to be perceived as useful and necessary design, and therefore, it is vital to keep users in mind when designing and offering DHCSs. On the other hand, people are profoundly different from each other, and this presents a significant obstacle in all system development initiatives. It is also easy to forget that many people have comorbidities and that each and every condition may manifest itself differently from one person to another.

DHCSs can undoubtedly support the achievement of different SDGs, especially SDG 3 related to ensuring healthy lives and promoting well-being for all at all ages. But to achieve that, digital competence is needed, and this varies from person to person affected by, for example, age or education level. To address these issues, DHCSs need to be reinforced by both non-digital options and digital health literacy training programmes. Additionally, since a person's health condition may be in constant flux, caregivers will continuously need to evaluate the adequacy of digital services offered and used by that person. Correspondingly, the DHCSs themselves should be subject to continuous evaluation and change, depending on for what and for whom the service is made and offered.

6.9 Relevance to Clinical Practice

The study provides valuable insights on how to develop DHCSs. DHCSs are important in developing sustainable healthcare services and for supporting patient-centred care, which are prominent topics in contemporary political and societal discussions on developing future healthcare services. DHCSs affect health services both from an organisational and an individual perspective, providing improved opportunities for communication and interaction between the patient and the healthcare services. Other examples may be the contribution of AI for faster and more accurate diagnostics, or using sensor technology that may enable a patient to stay at home and not be hospitalised. However, it should be kept in mind that to make use of the potential of DHCSs, patients and users need to gain a certain level of digital health literacy, which should be present both on an individual (user) and organisational level (caregiver). Thus, arenas for education and support are needed, and healthcare organisations should be aware of how their services are developed, which calls for joint interaction with developers, users, and organisations for creating future DHCSs.

Author Contribution The authors are listed alphabetically. All authors have contributed equally, albeit on different parts, to this chapter.

References

Adams T, Holman Jones S, Ellis C (2015) Autoethnography. Oxford University Press, New York

Anderson L (2006) Analytic autoethnography. J Contemp Ethnogr 35(4):373–395

Askheim OP, Andersen J (2023) Brukermedvirkningens mange ansikter (The many faces of user participation). Fagbokforlaget, Bergen. ISBN 978-82.450-4159-0

Birnbaum F, Lewis D, Rosen RK, Ranney ML (2015) Patient engagement and the design of digital health. Acad Emerg Med 22(6):754–756. https://doi.org/10.1111/acem.12692

Bjønness AM, Midtbø T, Størset H, Ulven CH (2021) Befolkningens digitale kompetanse og deltakelse. Med et ekstra blikk på seniorer og ikke sysselsatte. (The population's digital competence and participation. With an extra look at seniors and not employed). Kompetanse Norge. Report. ISBN 978-82-7724-383-2

Conquergood D (2002) Performance studies: interventions and radical research. TDR/Drama Rev 46(2):145–156

Creswell JW (2014) Research design. Qualitative, quantitative, and mixed methods approaches, 4th edn. Sage, Thousand Oaks

Dunn P, Hazzard E (2019) Technology approaches to digital health literacy. Int J Cardiol 293:294–296, ISSN 0167-5273. https://doi.org/10.1016/j.ijcard.2019.06.039

Ellis C, Adams TE, Bochner AP (2011) Autoethnography: an overview. Forum qualitative Sozialforschung/forum: qualitative. Soc Res 12(1):Art. 10. http://nbn-resolving.de/urn:nbn:de:0114-fqs1101108

European Union (2016) Directive (EU) 2016/2102 on the accessibility of websites and mobile applications of public sector bodies. https://eur-lex.europa.eu/legal-content/EN/TXT/?uri=CELEX%3A32016L2102. Accessed 20 Mar 2023

Førde R (2014) Helsinkideklarasjonen. De nasjonale forsknngsetiske komiteene (The declaration of Helsinki The national research ethics committees), Norway. https://wwwforskningsetikkno/ressurser/fbib/lover-retningslinjer/helsinkideklarasjonen/. Accessed 9 Dec 2023

Gerlach R (2019) Why should sustainability be an issue in digital health care? 4 ways digital health companies can help achieve sustainable development goals. https://wwwtbdcommunity/en/a/why-should-sustainability-be-issue-digital-healthcare. Accessed 4 Apr 2023

Halvorsen K, Jerpseth H (2016) Forskningsetiske utfordringer ved kvalitative studier (Research ethical challenges in qualitative studies). Sykepleien forskning, Oslo, p 57440

Helsedirektoratet (2020) Utredning av tilbud til hørselshemmede (Assessment of services for the hearing impaired). Oslo. Helsedirektoratet. https://www.helsedirektoratet.no/rapporter/utredning-av-tilbud-til-horselshemmede. Accessed 14 Feb 2023

Heponiemi T, Kaihlanen AM, Kouvonen A, Leemann L, Taipale S, Gluschkoff K (2022) The role of age and digital competence on the use of online health and social care services: a cross-sectional population-based survey. Dig Health 8:1–10. https://doi.org/10.1177/20552076221074485

Klevan TG, Sælør KT, Sundet R (2019) Ensretting, standardisering og kunnskapsbasert praksis – autoetnografi som motstand? (Alignment, standardization and knowledge-based practice – autoethnography as resistance?). Forskning&Forandring 2(2):105–123

Kvale S, Brinkmann S (2015) Det kvalitative forskningsintervju (Qualitative research interviewing), 3rd edn. Gyldendal Akademisk, Oslo

Nielsen J (1999) Designing web usability: the practice of simplicity. New Riders Publishing, Thousand Oaks

Norman CD, Skinner HA (2006) eHealth literacy: essential skills for consumer health in a networked world. J med internet res. Jun 16;8(2): e9. 8. https://doi.org/10.2196/jmir.8.2.e9

Palumbo R, Nicola C, Adinolfi P (2022) Addressing health literacy in the digital domain: insights from a literature review. Kybernetes 51(13):82–97

Santana S, Brach C, Harris L, Ochiai E, Blakey C, Bevington F, Kleinman D, Pronk N (2021) Updating health literacy for healthy people 2030: defining its importance for a new decade in public health. J Public Health Manag Pract 27(Suppl 6):S258–S264. https://doi.org/10.1097/phh.0000000000001324

Saunders M, Lewis P, Thornhill A (2019) Research methods for business students, 8th edn. Pearson Education Ltd., Harlow

Shah SHH, Longva B, Hameed IA, Solberg M, Hameed IA, Karlsen AST (2021) Health data Management for nursing practice: an intelligent, holographic mixed-reality system. In: Stephanidis et al (eds) Proceedings of the 23rd HCI (Human Computer Interaction) international conference, HCII 2021, CCIS 1420. Springer, Cham, pp 329–336

Shah SHH, Hameed IA, Karlsen AST, Solberg M (2022a) Towards a social VR-based exergame for elderly users: an exploratory study of acceptance, experiences and design principles. In: Chen JYC, Fragomeni G (eds) Virtual, augmented and mixed reality: design and development, HCII 2022. Lecture notes in computer science, vol 13317. Springer. https://doi.org/10.1007/978-3-031-05939-1_34

Shah SHH, Karlsen AST, Solberg M, Hameed IA (2022b) A social VR-based collaborative exergame for rehabilitation: codesign, development and user study. Virtual Reality 27:3403. https://doi.org/10.1007/s10055-022-00721-8

Shaw J, Agarwal P, Desveaux L, Cornejo Palma D, Stamenova V, Jamieson T, Yang R, Bathia RS, Bhattacharyya O (2018) Beyond “implementation”: digital health innovation and service design. NPJ Dig Med 1(48). https://doi.org/10.1038/s41746-018-0059-8

Smith B, Magnani JW (2019) New technologies, new disparities: the intersection of electronic health and digital health literacy. Int J Cardiol 292:280–282. https://doi.org/10.1016/j.ijcard.2019.05.066

Statistics Norway (2020) Et historisk skifte: Snart flere eldre enn barn og unge (A historic shift: soon more elderly than children and young people). https://wwwssbno/befolkning/artikler-og-publikasjoner/et-historisk-skifte-flere-eldre-enn. Accessed 4 Sep 2023

Statistics Norway (2022a) Allmennlegetjenesten (General practitioner services). https://wwwssbno/helse/helsetjenester/statistikk/allmennlegetjenesten. Accessed 14 Feb 2023

Statistics Norway (2022b) Digital sårbarhet: Hvem har høy risiko for å falle utenfor? (Digital vulnerability: who has high risk of falling outside?). Digital sårbarhet: Hvem har høy risiko for å falle utenfor? (ssb.no). Accessed 7 Sep 2023

Tjora A (2012) Kvalitative forskningsmetoder i praksis (Qualitative research methods in practice). Gyldendal Akademisk, Oslo

United Nations (2015) Transforming our world: the 2030 Agenda for sustainable development (A/RES/70/1). www.un.org. Accessed 19 Apr 2023

Vayena E, Haeusermann T, Adjekum A, Blasimme A (2018) Digital health: meeting the ethical and policy challenges. Swiss Med Weekly 148:w1457. https://doi.org/10.4414/smw.2018.14571

WAI (2016) Accessibility, usability, and inclusion. https://wwww3org/WAI/fundamentals/accessibility-usability-inclusion/. Accessed 10 Feb 2023

WCAG 2.1 (2018) Web content accessibility guidelines (WCAG) 2.1. The world wide web consortium (W3C) W3C recommendation 5th of June. https://www.w3.org/TR/2018/REC-WCAG21-20180605/. Accessed 10 Feb 2023

WHO (2021) Global strategy on digital health 2020–2025. World Health Organization, Geneva. 2021 License: CC BY-NC-SA 30 IGO. https://appswhoint/iris/bitstream/handle/10665/344249/9789240020924-engpdf. Accessed 11 Feb 2023

WHO (2023) Digital health. https://www.who.int/health-topics/digital-health/#tab=tab_2. Accessed 7 Apr 2023

Part III
Experiences of Care and Health Literacy

Chapter 7
Building Health Literacy: Health Professionals' Experiences in the Myocardial Infarction Pathway

Elise Kvalsund Bårdsgjerde, Bodil J. Landstad, Marit Kvangarsnes, Magne Nylenna, and Torstein Hole

Abstract This study aimed at exploring nurses' and physicians' experiences of building health literacy in the myocardial infarction pathway. A qualitative design was applied. Nurses participated in focus groups (n = 22) and physicians were individually interviewed (n = 9). The results are presented following the different phases of the myocardial infarction pathway with three distinct themes: precise and clear information (acute phase), starting to build health literacy (hospitalisation and discharge phase), and health-literate patients (rehabilitation phase). The findings showed that building health literacy varied depending on the different phases. The study revealed weaknesses in individual and organisational health literacy that require improvement. Health professionals participating in the study were concerned

E. K. Bårdsgjerde (✉)
Department of Health Sciences in Ålesund, Norwegian University of Science and Technology (NTNU), Ålesund, Norway
e-mail: elise.k.bardsgjerde@ntnu.no

B. J. Landstad
Department of Health Sciences, Mid Sweden University, Östersund, Sweden

Unit of Research, Education and Development, Östersund Hospital, Östersund, Sweden

M. Kvangarsnes
Department of Health Sciences in Ålesund, Norwegian University of Science and Technology (NTNU), Ålesund, Norway

Medical Department, Ålesund Hospital, Møre og Romsdal Hospital Trust, Ålesund, Norway

M. Nylenna
Institute of Health and Society, University of Oslo, Oslo, Norway

T. Hole
Medical Department, Ålesund Hospital, Møre og Romsdal Hospital Trust, Ålesund, Norway

Faculty of Medicine and Health Sciences, Norwegian University of Science and Technology (NTNU), Trondheim, Norway

T. Hole et al. (eds.), *Towards Sustainable Good Health and Well-being*,
https://doi.org/10.1007/978-3-031-61810-9_7

with preventing risk factors and promoting a healthy lifestyle. Cooperation between health professionals and organisations involved in the pathway must be improved to strengthen continuity in building health-literate patients. Promoting health literacy from a life span perspective is important for achieving Sustainability Development Goal 3: Good health and well-being, especially target 3.4, to reduce mortality from non-communicable diseases.

Keywords Myocardial infarction · Health literacy · Qualitative research · Sustainability Development Goals

7.1 Introduction

Health literacy empowers, drives equity, and has been positioned as a prerequisite for Sustainability Development Goal (SDG) 3: Good health and well-being. It is based on inclusive and equitable access to quality education and life-long learning (WHO 2017). Health literacy is an interdisciplinary and multidimensional concept involving individuals and organisations (Sørensen et al. 2012; WHO 2013; WHO 2017; Orkan 2019; Liu et al. 2020). Individual health literacy means the degree to which any individual/person can find, understand, and use information and health services to inform decisions and actions related to their health. Organisational health literacy is the degree to which organisations enable people to find, understand, and use information and healthcare services in decisions about their health and subsequent actions (Centers for Disease Control and Prevention (CDC) 2020). This understanding of health literacy involves a division of responsibility. Individuals are not solely responsible for strengthening their health literacy: healthcare organisations are expected to provide clear, accurate, appropriate, and accessible information (WHO 2017).

Several surveys have been developed to measure health literacy resulting in an amount of incomparable data measuring different variables, making it difficult to conduct valid systematic meta-analyses (Ghisi et al. 2018; Pleasant et al. 2019). The European Health Literacy Population Survey 2019–2021 (HLS19) of M-POHL has been developed to measure populations' health literacy in European countries (Pelikan et al. 2019). The first survey in Norway of the population's health literacy was carried out in 2018–2021 (The Norwegian Directorate of Health 2020). The survey showed that 33% of the population has low health literacy and may lack the key knowledge and skills necessary for self-care, avoiding risk factors or coping with disease treatment. No clear differences in health literacy between genders, age groups, level of education, or persons with and without long-term illness, were found (The Norwegian Directorate of Health 2020).

Myocardial infarction (MI) is a life-threatening condition that requires urgent medical and invasive treatment (Byrne et al. 2023). Patients with MI mostly have an underlying atherothrombotic process, which is a chronic condition caused by a combination of genetic, physiological, environmental, and behavioural factors

(Grovatsmark et al. 2020; WHO 2022; Byrne et al. 2023), and which can manifest itself through different acute and chronic diseases. Long-term treatment and lifestyle changes are required to control risk factors and reduce the risk of recurrent MI (Kotseva et al. 2016, 2019).

Acute MI is part of the acute coronary syndromes (ACS) spectrum. ACS are associated with a wide range of clinical presentations: from patients who are symptom free at presentation to prolonged chest discomfort/pain or cardiogenic shock or cardiac arrest. Patients presenting with suspected ACS are typically classified based on ECG results and the presence or absence of cardiac troponin elevation. Patients presenting with ST-elevation on their ECG are classified as having an ST-elevation myocardial infarction (STEMI), and patients without this ECG marker, who fulfil the MI criteria, as non-ST-elevation myocardial infarction (NSTEMI). The MI pathway differs for patients with STEMI and NSTEMI. Clinical guidelines and medical recommendations for the acute treatment of STEMI are important frame factors in the acute phase. The first choice of treatment is invasive, with percutaneous coronary intervention (PCI) within the first 120 minutes of medical contact (Byrne et al. 2023). Patients are treated with fibrinolysis followed by PCI when geographic distances prevent primary PCI within 120 minutes (Grovatsmark et al. 2020; Byrne et al. 2023). Invasive treatment is centralised in Norway; thus, ca. 50% of the patients are transferred between hospitals to receive treatment (Grovatsmark et al. 2020). In patients with NSTEMI, immediate or urgent PCI is recommended for high-risk patients within 24 hours, and delayed PCI is an option for patients not considered to be high risk (Byrne et al. 2023).

The treatment and care of MI (the MI pathway) can be divided into different phases, yet the phases often overlap (Bårdsgjerde 2022). In this research project, the MI pathway was divided into three phases: acute, hospitalisation and discharge, and rehabilitation. The acute phase starts at the point of first medical contact and ends with PCI treatment. The acute phase is followed by the hospitalisation and discharge phase; the final phase is rehabilitation. The rehabilitation phase consists of lifelong treatment supporting healthy lifestyle choices, optimising medications, and achieving and sustaining risk factor treatment targets (Byrne et al. 2023).

The treatment of MI should consider not only the best available evidence regarding clinical management but also the individual patient's preferences, needs, and values in clinical decision-making (Byrne et al. 2023). A person-centred approach improves patients' experiences of information, communication, and the involvement of family caregivers (Wolf et al. 2019) and might improve patient outcomes (Fors et al. 2017; Pirhonen et al. 2019). Involving and educating the patient are recognised as a key component in cardiac care and should take place throughout the MI pathway, from admission to hospital discharge and further into the rehabilitation phase (Byrne et al. 2023).

Patients with MI need sufficient health literacy enabling them to make multiple lifestyle changes and adhere to recommended medical treatment (WHO 2013). Studies have revealed that patients often experience insufficient information about their disease, lifestyle changes, and medications during the MI pathway (Decker et al. 2007; Pettersen et al. 2018; Bårdsgjerde et al. 2019; Valaker et al. 2020).

Patients' abilities to process, understand, and use health information might be reduced in acute situations (Astin et al. 2008; Svavarsdóttir et al. 2015).

A German study showed that over 40% of patients with cardiovascular disease reported difficulties in accessing, understanding, appraising, or applying health information in their daily life. In addition, the study identified that the largest differences between persons with and without cardiovascular disease were to understand health warnings about behaviours such as smoking, low physical activity, and use of alcohol and to judge which everyday behaviours is related to their health (Diederichs et al. 2018). A Norwegian-Danish study found that lower health literacy is associated with more behavioural and psychological risk factors in patients with cardiovascular disease (Brørs et al. 2022).

A systematic review suggested that the prevalence of low health literacy among these patients is, on average, 30%. It was identified that low health literacy led to increased re-admissions, lower quality of life related to health, increased anxiety levels, and a decrease in social support. Just one of the studies included in the systematic review investigated health literacy and its impact on cardiac rehabilitation (Ghisi et al. 2018).

Studies have shown that cardiac rehabilitation programmes reduce hospitalisation for cardio events, recurrent MI, and mortality caused by cardiovascular disease (de Araújo Pio et al. 2017; van Halewijn et al. 2017; Rea et al. 2020; Salzwedel et al. 2020; Dibben et al. 2021). In addition, meta-analyses have shown that patient education through cardiac rehabilitation leads to improved self-management behaviours (Aldcroft et al. 2011), increased health-related quality of life, and could potentially reduce healthcare costs (Brown et al. 2013; Dibben et al. 2021). This is supported by a systematic review demonstrating that educating patients increases patients' knowledge and behavioural changes regarding physical activity, diet, and smoking cessation (Ghisi 2014). An international concern is that the participation rate in cardiac rehabilitation programmes is low (Kotseva et al. 2016; Olsen et al. 2018; Norekvål et al. 2023).

The aim of this study was to explore nurses' and physicians' experiences in building health literacy in the MI pathway. The research question was:

How do nurses and physicians experience building health literacy in the myocardial infarction pathway?

7.2 Methods

7.2.1 Design

The study employs qualitative design using a thematic analysis method (Braun and Clarke 2006). A qualitative approach provides insight into health professionals' perceptions and experiences with the phenomenon of health literacy. Thematic analysis is a tool used to identify, analyse, and report patterns within the data. This tool is flexible in providing rich, detailed, yet complex, data (Braun and Clarke 2006).

Table 7.1 Demographic data

Participants (n)	Gender (F/M)	Age (average)	Education	Clinical experience in cardiac care in years (average)
22 nurses	19 F, 3 M	24–58 (37.8)	22 bachelor in nursing 9 specialised in cardiac care 2 specialised in intensive care nursing 1 Master's degree	1.5–33 (12.5)
9 physicians	4 F, 5 M	30–66 (40.8)	9 medical education 4 specialised in cardiology/ internal medicine 1 PhD	1–32 (11.1)

7.2.2 *Participants*

The study was approved by hospital management at two hospitals in Mid-Norway. Contacts at the hospitals helped to recruit participants.

Participants were selected by purposive sampling (Polit and Beck 2020). To ensure variation in the sample, contacts were requested to invite male and female nurses and physicians of different ages, educational backgrounds, and experiences (Patton 2015). The following inclusion criteria were applied: (a) nurses and physicians who worked in cardiac care and (b) with a minimum of 1 year of experience within cardiac care.

Twenty-two nurses participated in focus groups and nine physicians were individually interviewed. Demographic data are presented in Table 7.1.

7.2.3 *Data Collection*

Interview guides with open-ended questions were developed based on both the research question and previous research. The interview questions were related to providing information, for example, what information was provided during the different phases of the MI pathway, by whom, and in which way. Other questions were related to patient engagement and involvement, and how and when they were involved in their treatment and care. Follow-up questions were asked as appropriate.

Five focus groups with nurses and nine individual interviews with physicians were carried out from February to November 2018. The focus groups lasted approximately 90 minutes. The size of the focus groups varied from three to five participants. The individual interviews lasted between 27 and 58 minutes, with a mean duration of 43 minutes. The interviews were carried out by the first author; the third author co-moderated the focus groups. The interviews were audio-recorded and transcribed verbatim. Data saturation was achieved when we considered that the collected data were rich, and we could identify redundancies and patterns (Krueger and Casey 2015; Polit and Beck 2020).

7.2.4 *Ethical Considerations*

The Norwegian Centre for Research Data approved the study (Project number 56617). Written informed consent was obtained before data collection. Participants were informed that they could withdraw from the study without giving a reason. To avoid participant identification, demographic data and quotes applied in the results section cannot be linked to individual participants.

7.2.5 *Trustworthiness and Rigour*

The study was conducted in accordance to the Consolidated Criteria for Reporting Qualitative Research Guidelines (COREQ) (Tong et al. 2007). To ensure credibility, the methods and choices made are described in an explicit and transparent manner, and quotations were chosen to substantiate the results. At the end of each focus group, the co-moderator summarised the content, providing the participants with opportunities to add supplementary comments, to increase credibility. The analysis was performed by the first author. To achieve confirmability in the analysis, the co-authors read the transcripts, and the results were discussed. The results are presented through detailed descriptions enabling the readers to assess transferability (Lincoln and Guba 1985; Polit and Beck 2020).

7.3 Data Analysis

The data analysis was directed by both the research question and theoretical perspectives and earlier research on health literacy (Sørensen et al. 2012; Centers for Disease Control and Prevention (CDC) 2020).

In the data analysis, we followed the six phases described by Braun and Clarke (2006). In phase one, the interviews were read and re-read searching for meanings and patterns across them. In phase two, coding began. The data set was divided into three phases of the MI pathway: acute, hospitalisation and discharge, and rehabilitation. Initial codes were developed based on the different phases of the pathway. Extracts from the data set were chosen and labelled in the initial codes. When all data were collated into initial codes, the codes were analysed. We then considered how different codes could be combined to form overarching themes for each phase of the pathway. In the fourth phase, we reviewed the themes, and in phase five and six, the themes were defined, named, and written out in full. Quotations were used to underpin the results. Three themes were developed related to the different phases of the MI pathway.

The first author conducted the data analysis. The data analysis process and the development of sub-themes and themes were discussed by all authors. The data analysis was not a linear process but performed by a constant movement back and forth between the data set and the coded data extracts.

7.4 Results

The results showed how 22 nurses and 9 physicians experienced building health literacy in different phases of the MI pathway. The results are presented through three themes related to the acute phase, the hospitalisation and discharge, and the rehabilitation phase.

7.4.1 Precise and Clear Information: Acute Phase

Nurses and physicians expressed that for patients diagnosed with ST-elevation myocardial infarction (STEMI), it was necessary to convey concise and precise information to the patient about the diagnosis and what would happen: *"(By) then it is usually very urgent, so there is no time for a conversation, but we try to give concise information before we take them into the Angio Lab"* (Physician 1). They emphasised that it was important to reassure patients when carrying out life-saving treatment. During the acute phase, the nurses and physicians experienced that the patient often did not have the prerequisite knowledge to understand the overall picture of the disease: *"The patients know little about the disease and treatment. So, we cannot expect them to understand what is happening"* (Focus group 3, Nurse 1). Some of the participants worked at the Angio Lab and they said that they often had "a here and now focus" during treatment. A nurse stated: *"We tell them some basics while we're at it, we do what we have to do and provide information to the patient at the same time"* (Focus group 2, Nurse 2).

During the acute phase, the nurses and physicians reported that saving lives and carrying out the treatment was a priority rather than building health literacy. Experienced nurses conveyed that the acute phase could present *teachable moments*, where the patient wanted to learn about the disease: *"I think it is limited how therapeutic the information in the Angio Lab is, but the potential is there to guide them further"* (Focus group 2, Nurse 1).

The health professionals said that the transfer of patients between hospitals for PCI was often poorly planned for. For example, patients could be lacking personal belongings, such as clothes for the journey home, money, personal identification, and a mobile phone. This could cause problems for the patient upon discharge and their return home. It seems as if at an organisational level, health literacy was deficient in planning the patient pathway. There was a systemic lack of planning for the practical aspects of travel to, and from, PCI hospitals.

7.4.2 Starting to Build Health Literacy: Hospitalisation and Discharge

Nurses and physicians stated that patients with non-ST-elevation myocardial infarction (nSTEMI) received more information before the angiography and treatment. These patients were prepared with systematic information from physicians and nurses, both in oral and written form. Nurses and physicians emphasised that this information often had to be repeated, as it seemed to be difficult for patients to understand the complexity of the treatment intervention.

Patients were offered group education about the disease and control of risk factors. The nurses said that they emphasised which risk factors the patients themselves could influence, such as medication adherence, smoking cessation, physical activity, and diet. Health professionals experienced that patients were receptive to information and that an MI often presents *teachable moments* where patients were motivated to engage in building health literacy. Health professionals were aware that the pathway was short, which often led to challenges in the continuity of patient education. They conveyed that there was a need to systematise patient information in patient records. Information about whether the patient had understood the provided information was not documented: *"The documentation system we have is too poor, we do not know what information the patient has received"* (Physicians 1).

Nurses and physicians described that the MI pathway was fragmented, which resulted in little continuity in follow-up by health professionals. This meant that the patient often met different and new health professionals. Nurses and physicians said that they asked open-ended questions or asked the patient to "re-tell", or repeat back, information that they had received, so they could capture what the patient had received and understood from the provided information. Nurses also reported that there was a lack of written information. Paper-based brochures were replaced by digital information which was unavailable to some patients. These shortcomings might be interpreted as challenges for achieving organisational health literacy.

The health professionals said that before being discharged, the patients had a thorough conversation with the physician. Both oral and written information were provided. A physician conveyed it as follows: *"I emphasise the discharge conversations, because we address the central points there. To sort of summarize the whole hospital stay, provide good reasons for why you have started taking medication and the complete medication list, and how the patient should proceed. Patients with MI have very short hospital stays, and prior to discharge they need some time"* (Physician 6). The health professionals considered their patients' discharge as a good opportunity for building health literacy, and for empowering the patient to make good choices related to medications and lifestyle changes.

Both nurses and physicians expressed that it was difficult to communicate with patients who were not motivated to undertake cardiac rehabilitation, medication adherence, or lifestyle changes. Health professionals experienced a lack of resources and time to meet the extensive needs for motivation related to lifestyle changes and adherence to treatment in these patients. Nurses and physicians conveyed that they sometimes tried to involve family caregivers to motivate patients to, for example, participate in cardiac rehabilitation. It was a balance between motivating and persuading the patients: *"Sometimes we trick them into (undertaking) cardiac rehabilitation, but I think that is the best we can do for them"* (Focus group 3, Nurse 4).

7.4.3 Health-Literate Patients: Rehabilitation Phase

Nurses and physicians communicated that they considered it important that all patients participated in a cardiac rehabilitation programme. The overall aim of cardiac rehabilitation is to reduce the risk of recurrences and progression of heart disease.

Nurses and physicians also said that different approaches to learning were used. The cardiac rehabilitation programme consists of teaching individually and in groups, where family caregivers could participate. Group lectures were held by physicians, nurses, physiotherapists, and nutritionists and consisted of providing information about the disease, prevention of disease development, medication, and lifestyle preventive measures such as stopping smoking, dietary changes, and physical activity.

Nurses and physicians further emphasised that group training was an important part of the educational programme in cardiac rehabilitation. Training was important for them in order to master being physically active. Nurses and physicians expressed that it was important for patients to learn that physical activity was safe and important in relation to preventing negative disease development. Health professionals experienced that the community of practice with other patients motivated and improved patients' own health literacy. By participating in the community of practice, they gained motivation, knowledge, and the will to make good lifestyle choices for their own health.

Individual counselling was provided by both nurses and physicians. This counselling consisted of adjusting medication according to symptoms and adapting lifestyle changes to the individual patient's risk factors: *"We apply a form for risk factors, and then we point out what they can do to reduce risk factors. Some have several risk factors, while others have fewer"* (Focus group 4, Nurse 1). Nurses and physicians emphasised that they could not force patients to make lifestyle changes, but that they tried to motivate them by providing information about why they should, for example, stop smoking.

Nurses and physicians said that empowering patients was vital in building health literacy. They conveyed that it was crucial that the patients accepted their own responsibility for making good choices related to their health and well-being:

"The responsibility lies not only with the healthcare system, but everyone is largely responsible for their own health and acts themselves. We cannot do everything for them, there is a part that we can do and that only we can do, and then there is a part which only the patient can do" (Physician 5). Building health literacy is a prerequisite for enabling patients to take control of, and manage, their own disease.

7.5 Discussion

We found that building health literacy varied depending on the different phases of the MI pathway. During the acute phase, individual and precise information was highlighted to meet patients' needs. During hospitalisation and at discharge, nurses and physicians started to build health literacy to achieve good health and well-being. During the rehabilitation phase, nurses and physicians emphasised the importance of the patients' awareness of their potential for achieving good health and well-being through adherence to medication regimes and lifestyle changes. The study revealed weaknesses in individual and organisational health literacy that needed to be improved.

Health professionals in this study expressed that patients needed short and precise information about treatment during the acute phase. Lack of information during this phase leads to frightening experiences for patients (Bårdsgjerde et al. 2019). It is vital to increase health professionals' competence so that they understand the importance of clear and individualised communication during the acute phase of MI. Previous research supports this finding (Decker et al. 2007; Höglund et al. 2010; Valaker et al. 2017; Bårdsgjerde et al. 2019).

Health professionals described that *teachable moments* often occurred during hospitalisation. These moments, which occur naturally when people experience stressful life events, make people more receptive to developing knowledge and skills and to adopting risk-reducing health behaviour (Rowlands et al. 2019). Research has shown that many patients stop taking life-saving medication prescribed as secondary prevention after an MI (Pettersen et al. 2018; Bjoerklund et al. 2020; Lopez-Jimenez and Gersh 2020). It is therefore important that health professionals utilise these *teachable moments* to improve patients' health literacy and their understanding of adherence to taking medication, especially for long-term treatment. It requires in-depth knowledge to understand how medication can prevent the disease from developing. Patients need in-depth knowledge and a high level of health literacy to understand and assess the importance of compliance. In our study, the health professionals emphasised the importance of using the *teach-back* technique to assess patients' understanding of provided information. The *teach-back* technique has been proven as a valuable intervention for increasing health literacy regarding secondary prevention of cardiovascular disease (Beauchamp et al. 2022; Byrne et al. 2023). Health professionals need a comprehensive approach in order to plan, implement, and assess learning processes to build health literacy (Kvangarsnes et al. 2023; Kvangarsnes et al. in press). The European Society of Cardiology guidelines emphasise the importance of including the patient's perspective in treatment and care. The guidelines recommend person-centred care to ensure that patients' preferences, needs, and values are taken into account throughout the clinical pathway (Byrne et al. 2023). Studies have shown that a person-centred approach leads to satisfied patients and achievement of treatment outcomes (Fors et al. 2017; Pirhonen et al. 2019; Wolf et al. 2019).

This study revealed shortcomings in organisational health literacy in the clinical pathway of patients with MI. These included a lack of continuity in the short and fragmented pathway, lack of paper-based written information material, and poor documentation of information in patients' records. Previous research has similar findings, showing that it is challenging to achieve a seamless flow of information in treatment and care during the MI pathway (Valaker et al. 2020).

Using digital information requires access to digital devices and skills. Population surveys in Norway have shown that a substantial proportion of the population is well prepared to use digital health services. Nevertheless, older people, immigrants, people with long-term illnesses, and people with low levels of education still have inadequate digital skills (The Norwegian Directorate of Health 2020, 2021). Many patients need personal assistance to access equipment and navigate digital learning resources. Health professionals in our study expressed challenges in using digital information resources. The acute illness reduced some patients' abilities to absorb information, and most of the patients lacked the digital devices needed to apply digital health information.

This study showed that the short and fragmented MI pathway hinders building health literacy. Physicians experienced that the system for documenting patient information was poorly developed. We suggest the implementation of a unique medical record process which follows the patient throughout the pathway with a specific section for patient information/health literacy. This would benefit both health professionals and the patient in planning, implementing, and assessing health information and education. We think this will strengthen continuity in building health-literate patients.

The health professionals in our study reported that patients have good learning outcomes from participating in cardiac rehabilitation programmes, which is in line with earlier research (Brown et al. 2013; Ghisi 2014; Dibben et al. 2021). The cardiac rehabilitation programme employs a person-centred approach and a family perspective which create an environment which supports lifestyle changes and medication adherence. Support from family members has also been shown to be effective in increasing knowledge and improving physical activity (Beauchamp et al. 2022). Norwegian studies have shown worrying results regarding attending cardiac rehabilitation among patients after MI (Olsen et al. 2018; Norekvål et al. 2023). Geographical variations across the country are identified, and a call for action is needed to improve the follow-up care of MI patients (Norekvål et al. 2023).

Based on this study and previous research, we argue that building health literacy is important for achieving SDG 3 (Good health and well-being) for patients with heart diseases. Increasing patients' health literacy regarding medications and lifestyle changes after an MI may reduce mortality from non-communicable diseases, which is a specific target for SDG 3. Achieving this requires collaboration between health professionals, healthcare organisations at different levels, and patients and their family caregivers. This collaboration is thus linked to SDG 17: Partnership for the goals. Further research on health literacy and its effects on patients' good health and well-being is warranted.

7.6 Strengths and Weaknesses of the Study

Interviews with nurses and physicians provided a rich and nuanced understanding of health professionals' experiences with building health literacy during different phases of the MI pathway (Polit and Beck 2020). This provides new insight into how health professionals encounter patients' needs during the pathway. Nurses and physicians play a crucial role in building health-literate patients. The findings in our study are of great importance for the nurse and medical professionals involved in cardiac care.

We have not included data from a patient perspective in this study, which might be considered a weakness. Interviews with patients might have provided a more comprehensive understanding of the phenomenon of health literacy in the MI pathway.

The study was conducted in the context of health systems in Norway, which might also be a weakness regarding the transferability of the findings (Polit and Beck 2020). However, several of our findings could potentially be transferable to other countries with similar healthcare systems.

7.7 Conclusion

Building health literacy in the MI pathway is a joint responsibility, involving the individual patient, the health professionals, and the healthcare system. This study pinpointed the importance of utilising *teachable moments* during the pathway. Organisational health literacy should be developed to utilise those moments, and the health professionals must be aware of pedagogical tools to increase individuals' health literacy. Collaboration between health professionals and organisations involved in the pathway should be improved to achieve continuity in building health literacy. This study emphasised the importance of the cardiac rehabilitation programme to increase individual health literacy. These programmes have a person-centred approach and include the perspective of the family which is important for creating an environment supporting good health and well-being for the patients and their families. It will be important to assess the use of digital technologies in cardiac rehabilitation programmes in the future. Digitalisation of these programmes might not only be an important supplement to existing programmes but also an opportunity for patients who do not have access to cardiac rehabilitation programmes because of travel distances, work, or family obligations.

References

Aldcroft SA et al (2011) Psychoeducational rehabilitation for health behavior change in coronary artery disease: a systematic review of controlled trials. J Cardiopulm Rehabil Prev 31:273–281. https://doi.org/10.1097/HCR.0b013e318220a7c9

Astin F et al (2008) The information needs of patients treated with primary angioplasty for heart attack: an exploratory study. Patient Educ Couns 73:325–332. https://doi.org/10.1016/j.pec.2008.06.013

Bårdsgjerde EK (2022) Perceptions of patient participation in the myocardial infarction pathway among patients and healthcare professionals. Philosophiae Doctor. Norwegian University of Science and Technology (NTNU)

Bårdsgjerde EK et al (2019) Patient's narratives of their patient participation in the myocardial infarction pathway. J Adv Nurs 75:1063–1073. https://doi.org/10.1111/jan.13931

Beauchamp A et al (2022) Health literacy interventions for secondary prevention of coronary artery disease: a scoping review. Open Heart 9:e001895. https://doi.org/10.1136/openhrt-2021-001895

Bjoerklund E et al (2020) Secondary prevention medications after coronary artery bypass grafting and long-term survival: a population-based longitudinal study from the SWEDEHEART registry. Eur Heart J Open 41:1653–1661. https://doi.org/10.1093/eurheartj/ehz714

Braun V, Clarke V (2006) Using thematic analysis in psychology. Qual Res Psychol 3:77–101. https://doi.org/10.1191/1478088706qp063oa

Brørs G et al (2022) Health literacy and risk factors for coronary artery disease (from the CONCARDPCI study). Am J Cardiol 179:22–30. https://doi.org/10.1016/j.amjcard.2022.06.016

Brown JP et al (2013) Effect of patient education in the management of coronary heart disease: a systematic review and meta-analysis of randomized controlled trials. Eur J Prev Cardiol 20:701–714. https://doi.org/10.1177/2047487312449308

Byrne RA et al. (2023) 2023 ESC guidelines for the management of acute coronary syndromes: developed by the task force on the management of acute coronary syndromes of the European Society of Cardiology (ESC). Eur Heart J Open, ehad191. https://doi.org/10.1093/eurheartj/ehad191

Centers for Disease Control and Prevention (CDC) (2020) What is health literacy. Available https://www.cdc.gov/healthliteracy/learn/index.html. Accessed 28 Aug 2023

de Araújo Pio CS et al (2017) Effect of cardiac rehabilitation dose on mortality and morbidity: a systematic review and meta-regression analysis. Mayo Clin Proc, Elsevier 2017:1644–1659

Decker C et al (2007) Acute myocardial infarction patients' information needs over the course of treatment and recovery. J Cardiovasc Nurs 22:459–465. https://doi.org/10.1097/01.JCN.0000297391.11324.0f

Dibben G et al (2021) Exercise-based cardiac rehabilitation for coronary heart disease. Cochrane Database Syst Rev 2021. https://doi.org/10.1002/14651858.CD001800.pub4

Diederichs C et al (2018) Health literacy in men and women with cardiovascular diseases and its association with the use of health care services-results from the population-based GEDA2014/2015-EHIS survey in Germany. PLoS One 13:e0208303. https://doi.org/10.1371/journal.pone.0208303

Fors A et al (2017) Effects of person-centred care after an event of acute coronary syndrome: two-year follow-up of a randomised controlled trial. Int J Cardiol 249:42–47. https://doi.org/10.1016/j.ijcard.2017.08.069

Ghisi GLM et al (2014) A systematic review of patient education in cardiac patients: do they increase knowledge and promote health behavior change? Patient Educ Couns 95:160–174. https://doi.org/10.1016/j.pec.2014.01.012

Ghisi GLM et al (2018) Health literacy and coronary artery disease: a systematic review. Patient Educ Couns 101:177–184. https://doi.org/10.1016/j.pec.2017.09.002

Grovatsmark RES et al (2020) Norsk hjerteinfarktregister Årsrapport 2019 [The Norwegian Myocardial Infarction Register Annual Report 2019]. Available https://stolav.no/seksjon/Hjerteinfarktregisteret/Documents/%C3%85rsrapporter/%C3%85rsrapport%20 2019/2020-10-01%20Norsk%20hjerteinfarktregister%20-%20%C3%85rsrapport%20 2019_%20Innlevert_2.pdf. Accessed 21 Sep 2023

Höglund AT et al (2010) Patient participation during hospitalization for myocardial infarction: perceptions among patients and personnel. Scand J Caring Sci 24:482–489. https://doi.org/10.1111/j.1471-6712.2009.00738.x

Kotseva K et al (2016) EUROASPIRE IV: a European Society of Cardiology survey on the lifestyle, risk factor and therapeutic management of coronary patients from 24 European countries. Eur J Prev Cardiol 23:636–648. https://doi.org/10.1177/2047487315569401

Kotseva K et al (2019) Lifestyle and impact on cardiovascular risk factor control in coronary patients across 27 countries: results from the European Society of Cardiology ESC-EORP EUROASPIRE V registry. Eur J Prev Cardiol 26:824–835. https://doi.org/10.1177/2047487318825350

Krueger RA, Casey MA (2015) Focus groups: a practical guide for applied research, 5th edn. SAGE, Los Angeles

Kvangarsnes M, Dahl BM, Bårdsgjerde EK (2023) Helsekompetanse – en pedagogisk modell [Health literacy – a pedagogical model]. In: Dahl BM, Bjørnsen HN (eds) Helsesykepleie i praksis [Public health nursing in practice]. Fagbokforlaget, Bergen

Kvangarsnes M, Hole TL, Dahl BM, Landstad BJ, Bårdsgjerde EK (In press) Building health literary: A pedagogical model for good health and well-being. In: Hole TL, Kvangarsnes M, Bårdsgjerde EK, Landstad BJ, Tippet-Spirtou SE (Eds) Towards sustainable good health and well-being: the role of health literacy. Springe Nature

Lincoln YS, Guba EG (1985) Establishing trustworthiness. In: Lincoln YS, Guba EG (eds) Naturalistic inquiry, vol 9. Sage, Beverly Hills, p 438

Liu C et al. (2020) What is the meaning of health literacy? A systematic review and qualitative synthesis. Fam Med Commun Health 8:e000351. https://doi.org/10.1136/fmch-2020-000351

Lopez-Jimenez F, Gersh BJ (2020) Secondary prevention after coronary artery bypass grafting saves lives: a golden opportunity often wasted. Eur Heart J Open 41:1662–1664. https://doi.org/10.1093/eurheartj/ehz855

Norekvål TM et al (2023) Cardiac rehabilitation participation within 6 months of discharge in 37 136 myocardial infarction survivors: a nationwide registry study. Eur J Prev Cardiol zwad350. https://doi.org/10.1093/eurjpc/zwad350

Olsen SJS et al (2018) Cardiac rehabilitation after percutaneous coronary intervention: results from a nationwide survey. Eur J Cardiovasc Nurs 17:273–279. https://doi.org/10.1177/1474515117737766

Orkan O (2019) From Saranac Lake to Shanghai: a brief history of health literacy. In: Orkan O et al (eds) International handbook of health literacy. Policy Press, Bristol

Patton MQ (2015) Qualitative research & evaluation methods: integrating theory and practice, 4th edn. SAGE, Los Angeles

Pelikan JM et al (2019) Measuring health literacy in Europe: introducing the European health literacy survey questionnaire (HLS-EU-Q). In: Orkan O et al (eds) International handbook of health literacy. Policy Press, Bristol

Pettersen TR et al (2018) Challenges adhering to a medication regimen following first-time percutaneous coronary intervention: a patient perspective. Int J Nurs Stud 88:16–24. https://doi.org/10.1016/j.ijnurstu.2018.07.013

Pirhonen L et al (2019) Person-centred care in patients with acute coronary syndrome: cost-effectiveness analysis alongside a randomised controlled trial. Pharmacoecon Open 3:495–504. https://doi.org/10.1007/s41669-019-0126-3

Pleasant A et al (2019) Measuring health literacy in adults: an overview and discussion of current tools. In: Okan O et al (eds) International handbook of health literacy. Policy press, Bristol

Polit DF, Beck CT (2020) Nursing research: generating and assessing evidence for nursing practice, 11th edn. Lippincott Williams & Wilkins, Philadelphia

Rea F et al (2020) Better adherence with out-of-hospital healthcare improved long-term prognosis of acute coronary syndromes: evidence from an Italian real-world investigation. Int J Cardiol 318:14–20. https://doi.org/10.1016/j.ijcard.2020.06.017

Rowlands G et al (2019) Health literacy and chronic conditions: a life course perspective. In: Orkan O et al (eds) International handbook of health literacy. Policy Press, Bristol

Salzwedel A et al (2020) Effectiveness of comprehensive cardiac rehabilitation in coronary artery disease patients treated according to contemporary evidence based medicine: update of the cardiac rehabilitation outcome study (CROS-II). Eur J Prev Cardiol 27:1756–1774. https://doi.org/10.1177/2047487320905719

Sørensen K et al (2012) Health literacy and public health: a systematic review and integration of definitions and models. BMC Public Health 12:1–13. https://doi.org/10.1186/1471-2458-12-80

Svavarsdóttir MH, Sigurðardóttir ÁK, Steinsbekk A (2015) What is a good educator? A qualitative study on the perspective of individuals with coronary heart disease. Eur J Cardiovasc Nurs 15:513–521. https://doi.org/10.1177/1474515115618569

The Norwegian Directorate of Health (2020) Befolkningens helsekompetanse, del 1 [Health literacy in the Norwegian population, part 1]. Available https://www.helsedirektoratet.no/rapporter/befolkningens-helsekompetanse/Befolkningens%20helsekompetanse%20-%20del%20I.pdf/_/attachment/inline/e256f137-3799-446d-afef-24e57de16f2d:646b6f5ddafac96eef5f5ad602aeb1bc518eabc3/Befolkningens%20helsekompetanse%20-%20del%20I.pdf. Accessed 28 Aug 2023

The Norwegian Directorate of Health (2021) Helsekompetanse i fem utvalgte innvandrerpopulasjoner i Norge: Pakistan, Polen, Somalia, Tyrkia og Vietnam. Befolkningens helsekompetanse, del II [Health literacy in five selected immigrant populations in Norway: Pakistan, Poland, Somalia, Turkey and Vietnam. The Norwegian population's health literacy, part II]. Available https://www.helsedirektoratet.no/rapporter/befolkningens-helsekompetanse/Befolkningens%20helsekompetanse%20del%20II%20-%20Helsekompetansen%20i%20fem%20utvalgte%20innvandrerpopulasjoner%20i%20Norge.pdf/_/attachment/inline/10dec1b9-0d63-4746-ac27-041ed77238d0:372387142688ef9e57d78ba0f9b4a2f708f40746/Befolkningens%20helsekompetanse%20del%20II%20-%20Helsekompetansen%20i%20fem%20utvalgte%20innvandrerpopulasjoner%20i%20Norge.pdf. Accessed 28 Aug 2023

Tong A, Sainsbury P, Craig J (2007) Consolidated criteria for reporting qualitative research (COREQ): a 32-item checklist for interviews and focus groups. Int J Qual Health Care 19:349–357. https://doi.org/10.1093/intqhc/mzm042

Valaker I et al (2017) Continuity of care after percutaneous coronary intervention: the patient's perspective across secondary and primary care settings. Eur J Cardiovasc Nurs 16:444–452. https://doi.org/10.1177/1474515117690298

Valaker I et al (2020) Continuity of care and its associations with self-reported health, clinical characteristics and follow-up services after percutaneous coronary intervention. BMC Health Serv Res 20:1–15. https://doi.org/10.1186/s12913-020-4908-1

van Halewijn G et al (2017) Lessons from contemporary trials of cardiovascular prevention and rehabilitation: a systematic review and meta-analysis. Int J Cardiol 232:294–303. https://doi.org/10.1016/j.ijcard.2016.12.125

WHO (2013) Health literacy The solid facts. Available https://apps.who.int/iris/bitstream/handle/10665/128703/e96854.pdf. Accessed 28 Aug 2023

WHO (2017) Shanghai declaration on promoting health in the 2030 Agenda for Sustainable Development. Available https://www.who.int/publications/i/item/WHO-NMH-PND-17.5. Accessed 28 Aug 2023

WHO (2022) Noncommunicable diseases. Available https://www.who.int/news-room/fact-sheets/detail/noncommunicable-diseases. Accessed 21 Sept 2023

Wolf A, Vella R, Fors A (2019) The impact of person-centred care on patients' care experiences in relation to educational level after acute coronary syndrome: secondary outcome analysis of a randomised controlled trial. Eur J Cardiovasc Nurs 18:299–308. https://doi.org/10.1177/1474515118821242

Chapter 8
Patient Experience Following Lumbar Spinal Stenosis and Surgical Treatment

Liv Bakke, Marit Kvangarsnes, Vigdis Schnell Husby, Anne Lise Sagen-Major, and Erland Hermansen

Abstract The aim of the study was to gain insight into patient experiences following lumbar spinal stenosis and surgical treatment. Lumbar spinal stenosis is one of the most common diagnoses for surgical treatment worldwide, and the incidence is increasing. The most common symptoms of lumbar spinal stenosis are pain, reduced function, and reduced quality of life. The diagnosis has great costs for society and for the good health and well-being of both patients and their relatives. The study has a qualitative design. Purposive sampling was used, and nine in-depth interviews with open-ended questions were conducted in central Norway in 2018. The interviews were analysed according to Giorgi's phenomenological method. Four themes related to different phases of the clinical pathway were identified. The first and second themes express the way in which patients experienced their life situation

L. Bakke
Outpatient Pain Clinic, Møre and Romsdal Hospital Trust, Ålesund, Norway

M. Kvangarsnes (✉)
Department of Health Sciences in Ålesund, Norwegian University of Science and Technology (NTNU), Ålesund, Norway

Medical Department, Ålesund Hospital, Møre og Romsdal Hospital Trust, Ålesund, Norway
e-mail: marit.kvangarsnes@ntnu.no

V. S. Husby
Department of Health Sciences, Norwegian University of Science and Technology, Ålesund, Norway

Department of Orthopedic Surgery, Trondheim University Hospital, Trondheim, Norway

A. L. Sagen-Major
Norwegian University of Science and Technology, Ålesund, Norway

E. Hermansen
Kysthospitalet in Hagevik, Orthopedic Clinic, Haukeland University Hospital, Bergen, Norway

Department of Clinical Medicine, University of Bergen, Bergen, Norway

Møre og Romsdal Hospital Trust, Ålesund, Norway

T. Hole et al. (eds.), *Towards Sustainable Good Health and Well-being*,
https://doi.org/10.1007/978-3-031-61810-9_8

before surgical treatment; the third and fourth themes describe their experiences after treatment. The study found that patients had been in pain for many years and had experienced reduced participation in work and social life before the operation. Patients experienced a fresh start after the operation with full and productive employment. Achieving productive employment and decent work was experienced as important for good health and well-being (SDG 3 and SDG 8). The knowledge from this study is important for both patients and health personnel for creating health-literate individuals and organization for facilitating good health and well-being (SDG3). Knowledge about patient experience following lumbar spinal stenosis and surgical treatment should be included as a topic in the education of health personnel. Healthcare providers should offer the patients education programmes ahead of surgery ensuring environmental support and health-literate patients in the clinical pathway (SDG4).

Keywords Lumbar spinal stenosis · Orthopaedics · Patient experience · Clinical pathway · Good health and well-being · Productive employment · Health literacy

8.1 Introduction

Lumbar spinal stenosis is one of the most common reasons for lumbar surgery in older people over the age of 65 (Kovacs et al. 2011; Deer et al. 2019). Ravindra et al. found that the incidence of degenerative lumbar disease worldwide is estimated at 266 million (3.63%) individuals per year, with the highest incidences found in Europe (5.7%) (Ravindra et al. 2018). The diagnosis is one of the most common among spinal disorders and increases with age, with little difference in prevalence between sexes (Deer et al. 2019).

Lumbar spinal stenosis defines a narrowing of the spinal canal, leading to compression of the nerves and vessels in the spinal cord (Hermansen et al. 2017). It is caused by degenerative changes and causes clinical symptoms such as pain in the lower back, numbness, pain in the feet, especially when walking, and neurogenic claudication. The condition can also result in a reduced level of functioning due to pain. Little or moderate pain often leads to conservative treatment, and the assessment of the potential benefit of the operation should exceed any risk from surgical treatment (Nerland et al. 2015).

Nurses play an important role in providing care before, during, and after surgery. Knowledge about patients' lived experiences is important so that nurses can provide individually adapted information in the course of disease (Hébert et al. 2020). Nurses often meet patients at the outpatient clinic prior to operation. Preoperative instructions may affect patients` outcome of treatment and benefit own health (Carmona and Pleasant 2018). In an orthopaedic ward, nurses play an important role in providing nursing and treatment. The nurse is the team coordinator and will collaborate interdisciplinary and transdisciplinary with team members who will cover all the patients' needs, including all health services. It is crucial that patients receive sufficient information before surgery to maintain realistic expectations of treatment outcome and to strengthen their ability to master further rehabilitation after surgery (van der Horst et al. 2019). It is essential to improve patients` health skills to promote and provide good health and well-being (Sørensen et al. 2012, 2021; Gibney et al. 2020) and decent work for all which is central to economic and social progress and societal well-being (Di Ruggiero et al. 2015).

8.2 Background

Patients with symptoms of lumbar spinal stenosis experience back pain and articulating pain. In some cases, it can be difficult to make a specific diagnosis for this group of patients. The diagnosis is often based on the clinical symptoms with the corresponding findings of radiological investigations (Jensen et al. 2020). Many patients with lumbar spinal stenosis are offered surgical treatment. Posterior decompression is a collective term for multiple posterior decompression techniques used to relieve nerve compression in the spinal canal. These different techniques are used to create better conditions for the nerve structures of the spinal cord. This is created by removing deposits and surrounding tissues (Hermansen et al. 2017).

A survey conducted in the United States showed that surgical treatment of lumbar spinal stenosis led to a significant improvement compared with conservative treatment. Improvements in terms of pain and function were reported, and patients were more satisfied with their progression after surgery (Weinstein et al. 2010). Surgical treatment of lumbar spinal stenosis has also been reported to be superior to conservative treatment in terms of physical improvement. Patients with clinical symptoms of neurogenic claudication before treatment report remarkable improvement after treatment (Kovacs et al. 2011). Corresponding studies also show positive results considering both lower back pain and foot pain (Weinstein et al. 2010; Ikuta et al. 2016).

Several qualitative studies have explored patient experiences without surgical treatment for lumbar spinal stenosis (Weinstein et al. 2010; Ikuta et al. 2016). The results showed that the effects of medical care and exercise treatment were generally temporary (Bove et al. 2018). A recent longitudinal study showed that patients who exercised regularly before surgery had significantly less pain in the lower extremities after surgical treatment (Hébert et al. 2020).

A lack of health literacy is found among certain groups in society. Older people, people with low education and low social status have noticeably poorer health literacy before undergoing orthopaedic surgery (Sørensen et al. 2015). Lower health literacy is a significant factor associated with increased use of healthcare services and costs (Haun et al. 2015). Realistic information about surgery treatment and postsurgical expectations can lead to better mental preparation before surgery and improved sense of control (Conradsen et al. 2016).

Recent data from the Norwegian population show that 20% had difficulty considering what kind of health service they need. The patients were unsure if the health service would cover their needs and felt uncertainty in deciding which healthcare services they should choose (IS-2959 2021). Qualitative research on patient experiences following lumbar spinal stenosis and surgical treatment is scarce.

Our objective in this study was to achieve a deeper understanding of the patient's experiences in the clinical pathway. The aim was to explore patients' lived experiences with lumbar spinal stenosis and surgical treatment. The research question was: How do the patients experience lumbar spinal stenosis and surgery in the clinical pathway? Knowledge about this is important to create health-literate patients and organizations.

8.3 Design and Methods

A qualitative research design with a phenomenological approach was chosen as the most appropriate method to gain knowledge of the lived experiences of the patients (Polit and Beck 2017). In-depth interviews were used to collect data. The four-step method established by Amadeo Giorgi was applied (Polit and Beck 2017). The study adhered to the COREQ 32-item checklist for qualitative studies.

8.3.1 Participants

Purposive sampling was conducted (Polit and Beck 2017). Patients who had undergone surgery for lumbar spinal stenosis were selected. They had not benefitted from conservative treatment and had undergone a posterior decompression of the affected level of the spine. Exclusion criteria were patients with cognitive impairment and other criteria that could have an impact on outcome, reoperations, fixations, and disc hernia surgery.

Eleven participants were drawn consecutively from the Health Agency's register between 16 May 2017 and 31 October 2017. The participants had undergone surgery for the first time, comprising only decompression. One patient withdrew from the study due to inconvenience and another was excluded due to exclusion criteria. After nine interviews, the information was repetitive and redundant, and we considered the data saturated (Polit and Beck 2017). Four women and five men aged 61–79 years participated in the study (Table 8.1).

Table 8.1 Participants' characteristics

Female/Male	4/5
Age	
50–60	0
60–70	5
>70	4
Average age	
Female	67
Male	72
Civil status	
Married	7
Living alone	2
Social status	
Retired	7
Disabled	2

Table 8.2 Interview guide

1. Can you tell me about your situation before surgery?
2. How did you experience pain and mobility before surgery?
3. What information did you receive before surgery?
4. How did you experience pain and mobility after surgery?
5. How did you experience your life situation after surgery?
6. Do you have anything else you want to say?

8.3.2 Data Collection

Participants were recruited by phone by a contact person who was not involved in the study. Patients were recruited 3 months after they had undergone decompression surgery. Individual in-depth interviews were used for data collection. The first author conducted the interviews. At the start of each interview, written informed consent was obtained. The interviews were audio-recorded and took place in the participant's home or in the hospital 3–9 months after surgery. The interviews lasted between 60 and 90 min. Interviews were transcribed immediately after each interview. Data were collected until each theme was abundant and copious and was intended to be repetitive and redundant (Richards and Morse 2012). An open-ended interview guide was developed (Polit and Beck 2017) (Table 8.2).

8.3.3 *Ethical Considerations*

The study was carried out according to the principles of the Declaration of Helsinki (2013) and was approved by the Regional Committee for Medical and Health Research Ethics (2017/2372 REK: Central Norway) participants were told that participation was voluntary and that their anonymity would be protected. They were also informed that they could withdraw from the study at any time. Informed consent to participate and consent to publish was obtained in writing prior to the start of the study. The collected data were stored according to the Regional Committee for Medical and Health Research Ethics requirement for storage of sensitive research material. Patients are vulnerable to surgical procedures, and it is important to prepare them for any emotional reactions (Polit and Beck 2017).

8.3.4 *Data Analysis*

The analysis started immediately after the first interview and followed Amadeo Giorgi's four-step method (Giorgi et al. 1985). The first step was to read all the interviews to get a sense of the entire survey. The first author then identified and coded the units of meaning related to the experiences before and after treatment. The second step was to transform the raw data into individual phenomenological descriptions (Giorgi 2009). Individual descriptions were organized under related themes with the same meaning content (Giorgi et al. 1985). The third step was to search for the underlying meaning in the meaningful units through a reflective and analytical process (Giorgi 2009). Finally, we summed up the significance of each experience, summarized the hierarchically arranged knowledge, and formed stories that could be retold to describe the essence of the phenomenon studied (Giorgi et al. 1985). Analyses were conducted in collaboration with the co-authors.

8.3.4.1 Rigour

The researchers described the methodological decision explicitly and carefully to the patients to enhance trustworthiness. The first author, in collaboration with the second author, performed the analysis. The analysis was thoroughly discussed with co-authors who did not have the same proximity to the research field. The various stages of the analysis were carefully documented to achieve transparency in the research process (Polit and Beck 2017). To validate this process, three of the authors read the transcripts, and the findings were discussed with all authors.

8.4 Findings

Four women and five men described their experiences with lumbar spinal stenosis and surgical treatment in the clinical pathway. Four themes were identified: (a) like a red-hot iron rod towards the hip, (b) stopping meaningful activities, (c) rapid recovery from pain, and (d) having a fresh start.

8.4.1 *Like a Red-Hot Iron Rod*

Patients said that they had been in pain for many years. The pain was strong and constant and was described as "a glowing iron rod towards the hip" (Informant 1). Patients had experienced severe pain in both legs for 2–3 years before accepting surgical treatment. "The pain went especially over the hips, down the thighs when you touched them, but there was pain in the legs too" (Informant 6). One patient explained: "I had the feeling of something tight around the hip and most of the time I could not go very far in fear that my foot would fail" (Informant 8). Mostly, they had experienced pain during activity. The pain was located in the lower back and in one or both of the lower extremities.

Those who had experienced back pain felt a soothing effect when they sat or bent forward. Several of the respondents reported that they had experienced palsy in one or both lower limbs. They described it with words such as "tingling, pricking, and numbness". One patient described the experience as: "I felt like a knife stabbing my bottom, thighs, and sometimes I felt it somewhat all the way down to my ankles" (Informant 3). Another described the experience as: "I felt as the foot had withered away; it was living its own life" (Informant 7). Most experienced palsy in the bottom and thighs, some all the way down to their toes. This condition led to experiences such as instability: the foot would then give way and increased the tendency to falls.

8.4.2 *Refraining from Meaningful Activities*

The patients shared their experiences about personal consequences, such as reduced daily activities, less social participation, and the feeling of isolation. They described how living with constant pain had led to a reduced functional capacity and limited their daily life. One of the symptoms communicated was that the foot started to shake. A sense of stiffness and pain was described when starting any activity. This led to walking and taking small steps in fear that the foot would give way. Several had experienced occasional failure of one of the lower extremities. The patients described the functional limitations they had to face in daily life. Pain limited their ability to carry out daily activities; "it was not easy at any time, I asked my wife to help with things I could normally do by myself" (Informant 5). The patients felt compromised due to their dependence on the family to overcome daily tasks and activities. They felt a loss of identity and struggled with their self-confidence.

The patients said that they used crutches and were even supported by available fixtures at home while performing daily activities. They felt isolated; "for almost a year I couldn't do anything" (Informant 4). They were prevented from participating in recreational and family activities. One of the patients said that he could not drive his car. It was also difficult to walk. "I could only walk short distances before the pain started" (Informant 1). The patients described a walking distance of 200–300 meters, while for some it was even more limited.

The patients expressed that life before the operation was bad. They said that days were shortened due to poor sleep quality. Poor sleep quality often led to their early withdrawal from social activities. Some of the patients felt depressed due to the extensive limitations they experienced in their daily lives. Patients expressed how important their own motivation and willpower had been to overcome daily challenges. They experienced a loss of freedom. "I was mostly at home" (Informant 4). Patients explained that the limitations of daily life were the reason for choosing surgical treatment; "I felt useless and helpless" (Informant 3).

The patients said that prior to the operation, they had received useful information about the clinical pathway from health personnel during a day visit to the hospital. They had received information from the nurse, the orthopaedic, the physiotherapist, and the anaesthetic doctor. Some of the patients felt that they received a bit too much information in just 1 day.

8.4.3 Rapid Recovery from Pain

After surgery, the patients experienced rapid recovery from pain. They described an immediate change after treatment and some even experienced no pain even before leaving the hospital. "As soon as I woke up and was able to stand on my feet, I realized that I could not feel any pain. I cried, it felt fantastic, it was like being re-born" (Informant 4). The patients' narratives about surgical treatment were accompanied by smiles and gratitude. Some patients described gradual improvement. One of them declared that after 2 months he felt "free of pain" (Informant 1). However, another said that he could still feel pain. Most patients who had experienced paralysis and weakness of the lower extremities before the operation noticed a feeling of improvement immediately after surgical treatment. This was always the first improvement experienced and mentioned after surgery. Shortly after surgery, some respondents still experienced palsy in their toes, albeit to a much lesser extent.

After surgery, most patients described the situation as having improved. Among patients who had experienced an improvement in function, most could perform daily tasks and gradually resume leisure activities. A patient reported that after a year of isolation, he could go fishing daily, he shone during the conversation, and showed great pleasure in his new life situation. He described pain after surgery as "it is completely gone" (Informant 4). Another patient spoke about improvement as "after the operation I was free of pain," and after returning home, she reported "I am gardening and doing exactly what I want" (Informant 5). However, one of the patients reported that walking steps was still a challenge, because the muscles were still weakened due to prolonged immobility. Some experiences after surgery were also described as a less positive outcome. The experiences were described by a small improvement and with some uncertainty about the final results of treatment. "It's mostly like only when I sat down that I couldn't feel the stabbing pain" (Informant 10). During the conversation, the same patient revealed that there may have been other conditions that could influence the persistent pain in the legs after surgery, "yes, there were tight veins" (Informant 10). Pain after surgery was also described by "back pain and pain in the hips still feel the same as before surgery" (Informant 6).

8.4.4 A Fresh Start

After surgery, patients experienced rapid recovery, and improvement was spoken of in terms of "like getting a fresh start" (Informant 8). This quote illustrates how many patients experienced their situation after treatment. They experienced life as good compared to what it had been in recent years; "I can now walk several miles" (Informant 1). The patients said that although they had high expectations for the outcome of the surgery, they had not realized that the outcome would be so successful; "the expectations are absolutely fulfilled" (Informant 5). Patients spoke of the remarkable and strong contrast as they described their quality of life before and after surgical treatment. The new possibility to participate in family life and work: "now I work 100%, there is nothing to stop me" (Informant 3).

The patients said that they would have preferred to have received treatment at an earlier stage of the disease. Some patients said they had been depressed due to pain and loss of function "I felt depressed before the operation you might say" (Informant 3), and they described the experience of feeling isolated from society and family life; "I mostly stayed inside the house" (Informant 4); "had it not been for the painkillers I would not have been able to get out of bed" (Informant 4). Some patients had been offered surgery earlier during the course of the disease and regretted that they had declined the offer; "as I said, I made the mistake of postponing the operation" (Informant 1). The patients revealed that if they had anticipated the consequences of postponing the operation, they would have chosen to receive surgery treatment at an earlier stage.

The patients expressed that they had experienced a lack of information about the possible positive outcome of surgery earlier in the pathway. They conveyed that an earlier operation in the clinical pathway might have prevented long-lasting pain and suffering related to the disease.

8.5 Discussion

Phenomenological analysis provided information on the patients' lived experiences with lumbar spinal stenosis and surgical treatment in the clinical pathway. The analysis revealed that the patients had experienced strong and constant pain before surgery. The severe pain had prevented them from participating in family and social life. They expressed a feeling of loss of identity. After treatment, patients experienced rapid relief from pain and regained family, social, and working life. The patients described the experience of a fresh start. The study provides valuable knowledge that can contribute to reaching sustainability goals regarding health and well-being and productive employment.

In the present study, the patients revealed that they had experienced strong and constant pain that had marked their lives before surgery. This is in accordance with previous research. A qualitative study by Van der Horst et al. found that some patients reported preoperative pain as unbearable and had not been able to work for a long period. Patients with lumbar spinal stenosis experience prolonged pain in the back and numbness and pain in the lower extremities (van der Horst et al. 2019). Our study highlights the consequences for patients such as loss of identity and the inability to participate in meaningful activities. The pain had prevented them from maintaining their family and social life. They experienced a loss of identity and were unable to preserve their family role. The experience of being dependent on relatives in daily life could threaten their independence and integrity.

The present study shows that patients with lumbar spinal stenosis experienced a reduced functional level and a significant loss of functional capacity. Earlier research supports this finding. Pahl et al. (2006) revealed that lumbar spine disorders in general have a severe negative impact on patient physical health and that lumbar spinal stenosis leads to a reduced functional level with consequences such as absence from work and social participation (van der Horst et al. 2019). Our study shows that the loss of functional capacity of the patient had significant consequences for simple daily tasks and led to isolation and depression.

The study showed that some of the patients experienced depression due to their difficult situations and felt compromised. This is consistent with earlier research (Nerland et al. 2015). Earlier studies have found that people living with constant pain and a reduced level of function are significantly more prone to struggle with anxiety and depression. Holmes et al. reported that depression in patients with chronic pain is associated with decreased function, poorer treatment outcome, and major healthcare costs. Our study supports this finding. The experiences of the patients of depression and isolation had brought consequences such as poor self-image and loss of freedom. Successful treatment of depression will reduce pain and improve function and quality of life for patients with chronic pain (Holmes et al. 2013).

After surgery, patients experienced an improvement in their quality of life. They talked about regaining their independence and being able to participate in family and social life again. Both the level of function and the pain are factors that influence the quality of life of patients (Katz 2002; Rustøen 2001). Previous research supports the results of this study by confirming the experience of patients of improved functions after treatment (Nerland et al. 2015; Hermansen et al. 2017). In the present study, the patients expressed rapid recovery of pain and functional level after surgery. They described how their progress created new optimism.

Earlier research shows that surgical treatment for patients with lumbar spinal stenosis is not always associated with a significantly better clinical outcome (van der Horst et al. 2019). A study by Hebert et al. highlights several potential predictors that have an impact on the outcome. They found that preoperative therapies and regular exercise were an important predictor of clinical outcomes (Hébert et al. 2020). Conradsen et al. highlight the importance of supporting patients with sufficient information before surgery to promote patients' ability to master their treatment decisions. Today, patients have access to a lot of information about their disease. Despite the amount of information, the interpretation of the information greatly depends on the reader's ability to fully understand its content and act on it. Health literacy is an important aspect of empowerment, which enables patients to make the best choices for their health (Conradsen et al. 2016). Health literacy consists of finding, understanding, accessing, applying, appraising, and using information about health to ensure one's own health (Sørensen et al. 2012, 2021). Recent data from the Norwegian population show that 20% had difficulty considering what kind of health service they need if the health service will cover their needs and to decide which healthcare services they should choose (IS-2959 2021).

Some patients said that they had experienced major consequences of the disease before treatment. Pain is associated with high costs for the healthcare system and society. Surgery treatment should be considered as an option earlier in the pathway when considering patients' treatment offers for this disease (Katz 2002; Holmes et al. 2013). The current study highlights the importance of patients having the necessary knowledge in the course of the disease to enable them to make knowledge-based decisions when considering treatment options for their disease. Navigating complex healthcare systems might be a major challenge when choosing different treatment options. Healthcare providers should be trained in a person-centred approach to meet individuals' needs. Health literacy sensitivity should be a quality criteria for health management and health professionals (Kickbush et al. 2013). This requires a focus in professional education and health personnel who are trained to communicate more effectively to meet the needs of patients with limited health literacy (Sørensen et al. 2012).

Our study revealed that most patients had experienced relief from pain and an increase in function after surgery. They expressed the importance of regaining their family role and being part of society. There was also a desire to receive surgical treatment earlier in the course of the disease. It is important that this knowledge be distributed to other patients so that they have the opportunity to make informed decisions before receiving treatment. Health personnel, together with their health trust, should undertake the responsibility to provide this knowledge. Social support and information from healthcare providers with good communication skills may lead patients to receive treatment for their disorders earlier in the disease (Bove et al. 2018). More qualitative research is needed to obtain wider knowledge about patients' experiences of various types of back surgery.

8.5.1 *Strength and Limitations*

A limited number of patients participated in the study; however, rich and detailed data were obtained. The results are likely to be transferable to other patients with a similar diagnosis, surgical treatment, and healthcare options (Polit and Beck 2017). Participants were recruited by staff not related to the study. Two of the interviews were conducted in the hospital, but the setting did not influence the willingness to share experiences. The verbatim transcription of the collected data was done by the first author immediately after each interview. The transcription was performed with great accuracy. The researcher's decisions are carefully documented to achieve transparency in the research process (Polit and Beck 2017). Two of the authors had professional positions close to the topic being studied. It was, therefore important to discuss the analysis with the co-authors who did not have the same proximity to the research field (Polit and Beck 2017).

8.6 Conclusion

The study has provided new knowledge about the patient's experiences of lumbar spinal stenosis and surgical treatment. The study showed that the patients had major pain ahead of surgery that stopped them from participating in meaningful activities. After surgery, patients experienced rapid recovery from pain and a feeling of a fresh start.

Advanced knowledge of patients` experiences is important when supervising patients to promote good health and well-being (SDG 3). This knowledge should be a theme in nursing and medical education as health personnel are responsible for supervising these patients in enhancing good health and well-being (SDG4).

It is important to strengthen a patient's personal health literacy to support the patient's decision-making process when considering treatment options and thus empower the patients in the clinical pathway. Health-literate patients are able to make sustainable and good choices for their own health (Gibney et al. 2020). Health literacy is equally important at an organizational level. Organizational health literacy is how organizations support individuals to find, understand, and use information and services to inform health-related decisions and actions for themselves and others.

References

Bove AM, Lynch AD, Ammendolia C et al (2018) Patients' experience with nonsurgical treatment for lumbar spinal stenosis: a qualitative study. Spine J 18:639–647

Carmona R, Pleasant A (2018) Becoming literate in health literacy. JAMA Surg 153:143

Conradsen S, Gjerseth MM, Kvangarsnes M (2016) Patients' experiences from an education programme ahead of orthopaedic surgery—a qualitative study. J Clin Nurs 25:2798–2806

Deer T, Sayed D, Michels J et al (2019) A review of lumbar spinal stenosis with intermittent neurogenic claudication: disease and diagnosis. Pain Med 20:S32–s44

Di Ruggiero E, Cohen JE, Cole DC et al (2015) Competing conceptualizations of decent work at the intersection of health, social and economic discourses. Soc Sci Med 133:120–127

Gibney S, Bruton L, Ryan C et al (2020) Increasing health literacy may reduce health inequalities: evidence from a national population survey in Ireland. Int J Environ Res Public Health 17:5891

Giorgi A (2009) The descriptive phenomenological method in psychology: a modified Husserlian approach. Pennsylvania, Duquesne University Press, Pittsburgh

Giorgi A, Aanstoos C, Fisher WF et al (1985) Phenomenology and psychological research. Duquesne University Press, Pittsburgh

Haun JN, Patel NR, French DD et al (2015) Association between health literacy and medical care costs in an integrated healthcare system: a regional population based study. BMC Health Serv Res 15:249

Hébert JJ, Abraham E, Wedderkopp N et al (2020) Preoperative factors predict postoperative trajectories of pain and disability following surgery for degenerative lumbar spinal stenosis. Spine (Phila Pa 1976) 45:E1421–e1430

Hermansen E, Austevoll IM, Romild UK et al (2017) Study-protocol for a randomized controlled trial comparing clinical and radiological results after three different posterior decompression techniques for lumbar spinal stenosis: the Spinal Stenosis Trial (SST) (part of the NORDSTEN Study). BMC Musculoskelet Disord 18:121

Holmes A, Christelis N, Arnold C (2013) Depression and chronic pain. Med J Aust 199:S17–S20

Ikuta K, Masuda K, Tominaga F et al (2016) Clinical and radiological study focused on relief of low back pain after decompression surgery in selected patients with lumbar spinal stenosis associated with grade I degenerative spondylolisthesis. Spine (Phila Pa 1976) 41:E1434–e1443

Is-2959 R (2021) The health literacy of the population, part 1. HLS19-rapport_Befolkningens helsekompetanse [The health competence of the population] del I. The Norwegian directorate of health

Jensen RK, Jensen TS, Koes B et al (2020) Prevalence of lumbar spinal stenosis in general and clinical populations: a systematic review and meta-analysis. Eur Spine J 29:2143–2163

Katz N (2002) The impact of pain management on quality of life. J Pain Symptom Manag 24:S38–S47

Kickbush I, Pelikan JM, Apfel F et al (2013) Health literacy. The solid facts. World Health Organization

Kovacs FM, Urrútia G, Alarcón JD (2011) Surgery versus conservative treatment for symptomatic lumbar spinal stenosis: a systematic review of randomized controlled trials. Spine (Phila Pa 1976) 36:E1335–E1351

Nerland US, Jakola AS, Solheim O et al (2015) Minimally invasive decompression versus open laminectomy for central stenosis of the lumbar spine: pragmatic comparative effectiveness study. BMJ 350:h1603

Pahl MA, Brislin B, Boden S et al (2006) The impact of four common lumbar spine diagnoses upon overall health status. Spine J 6:125–130

Polit DF, Beck CT (2017) Nursing research: generating and assessing evidence for nursing practice. Wolters Kluwer, Philadelphia

Ravindra VM, Senglaub SS, Rattani A et al (2018) Degenerative Lumbar spine disease: estimating global incidence and worldwide volume. Global Spine J 8:784–794

Richards L, Morse JM (2012) Readme first for a user's guide to qualitative methods. Sage, Los Angeles

Rustøen T (2001) Håp og livskvalitet : en utfordring for sykepleieren? [Hope and quality of life: a challenge for the nurse?]. Oslo, Gyldendal akademisk

Sørensen K, Van Den Broucke S, Fullam J et al (2012) Health literacy and public health: a systematic review and integration of definitions and models. BMC Public Health 12:80

Sørensen K, Pelikan JM, Röthlin F et al (2015) Health literacy in Europe: comparative results of the European health literacy survey (HLS-EU). Eur J Pub Health 25:1053–1058

Sørensen K, Levin-Zamir D, Duong TV et al (2021) Building health literacy system capacity: a framework for health literate systems. Health Promot Int 36:i13–i23

Van Der Horst AY, Trompetter HR, Pakvis DFM et al (2019) Between hope and fear: a qualitative study on perioperative experiences and coping of patients after lumbar fusion surgery. Int J Orthop Trauma Nurs 35:100707

Weinstein JN, Tosteson TD, Lurie JD et al (2010) Surgical versus nonoperative treatment for lumbar spinal stenosis four-year results of the spine patient outcomes research trial. Spine (Phila Pa 1976) 35:1329–1338

World Medical Association (2013) World Medical Association Declaration of Helsinki ethical principles for medical research involving human subjects. Available https://www.wma.net/policies-post/wma-declaration-of-helsinki-ethical-principles-for-medical-research-involving-human-subjects/. Accessed 11 Sept 2024

Chapter 9
A Narrative of Outsiderness: Visually Impaired Individuals' Experiences of Learning and Participation in Education and Working Life

Bodil J. Landstad, Gunhild Hovden Kvangarsnes, Stig Larsson, and Emma Brulin

Abstract This chapter deals with visually impaired individuals' experiences of learning and participation in education and working life. Health literacy is important at an individual and organisational level aiming at eliminating barriers and promoting equal opportunities for the visually impaired (SDG 10: Reduced inequality within and among countries). This study reveals that visually impaired individuals experience outsiderness in education and working life. The study also demonstrates the challenges and opportunities in participating in education and working life for the visually impaired in the future. The study provides important knowledge on how to strengthen good health and well-being (SDG 3: Good health and well-being) and promote quality education and life-long learning opportunities for the visually impaired (SDG 4: Quality education).

Keywords Visually impaired · Narrative · User experience · Health literacy · Adapted study resources · Digitalisation · Equal opportunities · Good health and well-being · Education · Working life

---

B. J. Landstad (✉)
Department of Health Sciences, Mid Sweden University, Östersund, Sweden

Unit of Research, Education and Development, Östersund Hospital, Östersund, Sweden
e-mail: bodil.landstad@miun.se

G. H. Kvangarsnes
The National Library of Norway, Oslo, Norway

S. Larsson
Department of Clinical Research, Lund University, Malmö, Sweden

E. Brulin
The Department of Occupational Medicine, Institute of Environmental Medicine, Karolinska Institute, Stockholm, Sweden

T. Hole et al. (eds.), *Towards Sustainable Good Health and Well-being*,
https://doi.org/10.1007/978-3-031-61810-9_9

9.1 Introduction

Visual impairment can be a hindrance to learning and participation in education and working life. This might lead to major personal problems and prevent people from becoming fully fledged members of society and working life. It is important to gain knowledge about how to facilitate participation for the visually impaired in various communities of practice during the life course. Communities of practice are defined as:

> groups of people who share a concern or a passion for something they do and learn how to do it better as they interact regularly. (Wenger 2011)

The aim of the following study was to explore experiences of participation. One of the authors has a visual impairment and thus provides a unique experience on the topic. At the same time, he is a researcher, a politician, and an engaged family father. He has contributed with data to this study, while also being a co-researcher. Being an active partner in the study may represent challenges that will be thoroughly discussed in the method section (Shippee et al. 2013; Kylberg et al. 2018). We have chosen a narrative approach because this methodology is appropriate for studying the life course perspective where the researchers are co-creators (Patton 2015).

9.2 Background

Visual impairment often results in significant disability and is associated with a substantial economic burden, reduced quality of life, medical issues, and loneliness (Gordois et al. 2012; Khorrami-Nejad et al. 2016; Dhital et al. 2010; Brunes et al. 2019). A review from 2020 concludes that considerable data indicate a high prevalence of depression and anxiety among people with visual impairments (Demmin and Silverstein 2020). Visually impaired individuals' experiences of unpleasant social situations or exclusion often result in insecurity, worry, avoidance, inactivity and social withdrawal, and depression (The Norwegian Association of the Blind 2023).

Access to text, literature, and e-books is important in order for the visually impaired to become full members of the community of practice. The national coordinator of accessibility of higher education in Norway and the Norwegian Library of Talking Books and Braille (NLB) have pointed to the fact that a large proportion of students have a disability that makes it difficult to read printed text or text presented in the form of images. Despite the increasing degree of digitalisation, there is very limited access to available digital versions of study literature that these students can make use of (The Norwegian Library of Talking Books and Braille 2017).

In a survey, carried out by the Swedish Council for Higher Education (2015), 17% of Swedish university students reported that they had a disability. Two-thirds of these students believed that the disability had hindered them in their studies.

Among the students reporting impaired sight or hearing as their disability, half of the students found their disability to be an obstacle in their studies (Swedish Council for Higher Education 2015).

The Swedish Agency for Accessible Media (MTM) is responsible for supplying academic literature to college and university students with a reading impairment. University libraries are the link between MTM and the student. All students with a reading disability can contact their university library, order an adapted version of their course literature, and borrow it in the form of a talking book, braille book, or e-textbook (The Norwegian Library of Talking Books and Braille 2017).

In Norway, only students with visual impairment have the right to order adapted study literature from the library service, NLB, provided by the National Library of Norway. Students with other reading disabilities can only lend adapted literature that already exists in the library. A Norwegian research report shows challenges in the requirement for a universal design of digital teaching aids in the university sector. Legal, economic, practical, and knowledge challenges are described (Proba Research 2019).

Research has shown that study fields such as chemistry, physics, engineering, biology, and mathematics have not been made easily accessible to blind and visually impaired students (Sahin and Yorek 2009). To learn science and mathematics, other senses such as touching and hearing are needed. The researchers concluded that classrooms should be adapted, and instruction should be adjusted for better science teaching to visually impaired students. They needed more tactile and audio experiences than visual instruction.

Access to English curriculum literature is important in education in Nordic countries. The agreement through the Accessible Books Consortium (2023) enables the exchange of adapted literature between countries. This means that a book produced in an adapted version in one country can be used by people in the target group in another country. The agreement is based on the owner of the rights agreeing that a title can be exchanged. The owner of the rights could say no to exchange without providing any reason. This situation is resolved through the Marrakesh Treaty (2013). The treaty states that a person who, due to functional impairment, has difficulty reading printed text has right to access adapted literature from all countries that have ratified the treaty.

A systematic review on the effect of assistive technology on the employment of individuals with visual impairment found that access to, and utilization of, assistive technology can help break down barriers and enable employment for blind and visually impaired workers (Ganz et al. 2020).

A British researcher, French (2017), has provided a deeper understanding of visually impaired people, their working lives, and their experiences of employment. She interviewed those who have worked in traditional jobs such as telephony, physiotherapy and piano tuning, and those who had pursued more unusual occupations. She grouped them according to occupation and framed them in a broader political, economic, ideological, and cultural context. The stories became an important part of policy work to facilitate participation in work in a group with high rates of unemployment. The user perspective is important for developing health services in accordance with user preferences.

Knowledge about visually impaired people's experiences of participation in education and working life is crucial to facilitate a health-literate environment. Health literacy is often defined on two levels: personal and organisational (Centers for Disease Control and Prevention 2020). Emphasis on health literacy at the individual and organisational level is of great importance for the visually impaired as the literature review shows that they have major challenges in participation in education and working life. Health literacy at both levels is paramount to reach the Sustainability Development Goal of good health and well-being (SDG 3), quality education (SDG 4), and reduced inequalities (SDG 10).

9.3 Theoretical Perspective

Theory about participation in the community of practice may give insight into visually impaired individuals' experiences of education and working life regarding learning, meaning, and identity.

The importance of revealing the researchers' underpinning thoughts and theoretical assumptions in narrative inquiry has been emphasized by Chase (2018). In this study, we considered a social constructivist approach to methodology and learning to be appropriate (Patton 2015; Wenger 2004), and a narrative approach was chosen (Patton 2015).

9.3.1 Learning

We have chosen "learning in communities of practice" as a theoretical framework in the interpretation of the storyline (Wenger 2004). Engagement in social practice is the fundamental process by which we know what we know and by which we become who we are. The theory explores the intersection of issues of community, social practice, meaning, and identity. Learning is a process of social participation and an encompassing process of being active participants in the practices of social communities and constructing identities. The communities of practice to which we belong change over the course of our lives.

Wenger (2004) states that in communities of practices, there are various types of trajectories: peripheral trajectories, inbound trajectories, insider trajectories, boundary trajectories, and outbound trajectories. Some trajectories lead away from communities, while others lead to becoming full participants in its practice. The trajectory has a coherence through time that connects the past, the present, and the future. A historical approach gives us ways of sorting out what is important, what contributes to our identity, and what is not important. Building identity is an ongoing process produced within a rich and complex set of relations of practice. Wenger (2004) describes identity as lived, negotiated, social, a learning process, a nexus, and a local-global interplay. The link between individual engagement and the formation of communities of practice is, according to Wenger, essential to a basic understanding of identity.

9.4 Aim

The aim of the study was to explore the visually impaired people's experiences of learning and participation in education and working life by creating a narrative representing experiences from different phases of their life course.

9.4.1 Method

We used a qualitative design (Patton 2015) with a narrative approach (Brinkmann and Kvale 2015). According to Brinkmann and Kvale (2015), a narrative can be based on stories from one or more persons. In this study, we have chosen to use one participant. The purposive sampling was based on the participants' unique experiences and insights in the field that was studied. His age, profession, and engagement in society gave rich and thick data. He had a position in the study both as interviewee and as co-author (Shippee et al. 2013; Kylberg et al. 2018).

9.4.2 Ethical Considerations

This study does not require ethical approval from the Swedish Ethics Authority because the interviewee is a co-author, but it requires informed consent (The Swedish Code of Statutes 2003:460 2005). We emphasized the building of reciprocal relationships and discussed our roles during the research process (Shippee et al. 2013). The interviewee has been involved in all parts of the research process—from the planning of the study to the published chapter. He has given a written consent to share his life story and experiences and to the use of personal data in the study and raised no objections from an ethical point of view. He has also given a written consent for the picture used in the analyses to be published. The interviewee was informed about his option to withdraw from the study without giving reasons.

The interviewee has generously shared his personal experiences, and we are aware that it can be perceived as burdensome (Kylberg et al. 2018). We have had a good dialogue about this throughout the research process, and he has expressed his satisfaction at being able to share his experiences and being a co-author. He has also expressed that he sees this contribution as very important for developing knowledge about a topic that is sparsely researched.

The project was carried out with the help of ethical guidelines according to the Declaration of Helsinki. This is a statement of ethical principles for medical research involving human subjects, including research on identifiable human material and data (World Medical Association 2013). The data were stored according to the Swedish Act on Ethical Review of Research Involving Humans (The Swedish Code of Statutes 2003:460 2005).

9.5 Data Material

We used different data sources to construct the narrative: a recorded radio interview, a private photograph, and individual interviews.

Radio Interview
The radio interview was conducted with the Interviewee in December 2012 at the International Disability Day where he talked about the exclusion disabled people have lived with throughout history (Swedish Radio—P4 Halland 2012). The interview was 4 min and 15 s long and is available online as an open-access resource.

Photograph
We used a photograph from 1998 taken in Berlin where the first author and the interviewee met at a conference on rehabilitation medicine. The photograph is from an evening event on the first day of the conference, in the beautiful ballroom in Das Rote Rathaus (the Town Hall). The event was held as an official welcome to the conference and a "get-together" for all the participants attending the conference. One common intention with these gatherings is that the participants meet in a relaxed manner and hopefully find new "research friends"—and thus expand their networks (Fig. 9.1).

Individual Interview
We interviewed one participant, Stig Larsson, three times in Spring 2023. He was born in 1943 with severe myopia (near-sightedness) but became increasingly visually impaired in his teens when he suffered from additional eye diseases. He is now almost completely blind and can only see (some) contours in the landscape. He is qualified as a professional social worker and qualified as a Doctor in Sociology in 1983. In 1992, he became a Professor in Social development and in 1997, Director of a Centre for Disability and Rehabilitation Research at Lund University in Sweden. When conducting this study, he was Professor Emeritus at the Department of Social Medicine and Global Health at Lund University.

We conducted three interviews via Teams in February and March 2023. The first two interviews were 2 h long, respectively, and the third was 1 h long. The first two interviews were carried out by the first and the second authors and, the third interview by the second author. All interviews were videotaped.

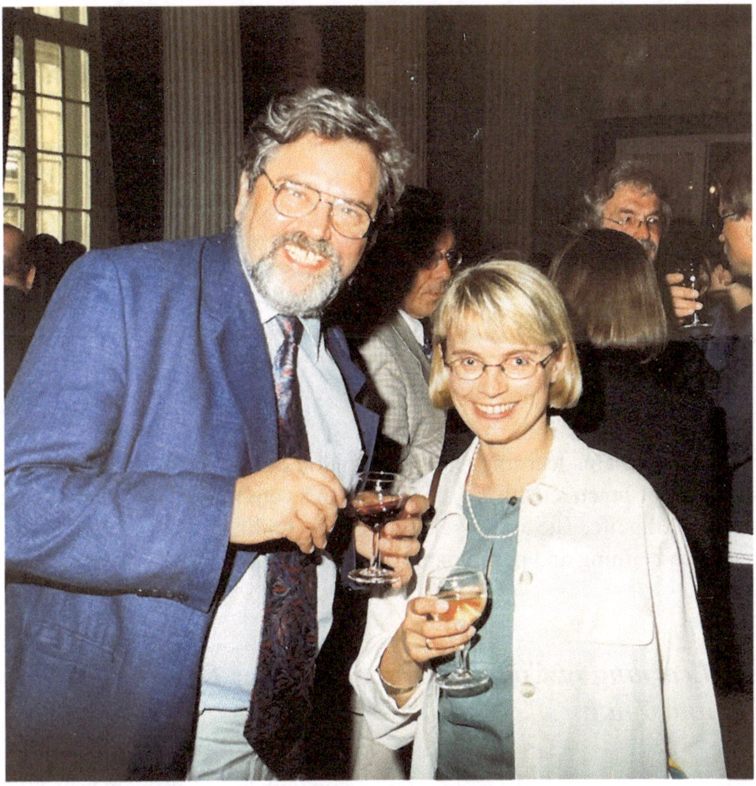

Fig. 9.1 Larsson and Landstad, Berlin 1998. (Photo: Author's own)

We used an interview guide with open-ended questions on childhood, adolescence, education, working life, and the future. The questions were about how visually impairment impacted participation in social life, education, and working life.

9.5.1 Analyses

When analysing the data, we used an inductive approach, with a focus on the narrative plot (Holloway and Freshwater 2007). First, we gained a holistic impression when looking at the photograph and listening to the radio interview and the informant interviews several times (Brinkmann and Kvale 2015). Meaningful units were identified and coded in relation to childhood and the period of adolescence, study time, working life, and plans for the future, all guided by narrative theory. By using a narrative approach (Holloway and Freshwater 2007), focusing on content, form, and context in the storyline of the interview, themes were identified for each phase, and the story was subsequently organized into a chronological structure (Patton 2015). Themes were created by organising the data into increasingly more abstract units. When analysing, we worked back and forth between the data and the themes until we had a comprehensive understanding of the data (Creswell and Creswell 2018). The interviewee, who also was a co-author, made significant contributions throughout the entire research process. Different professional backgrounds were important in the research group when interpreting relevant themes. Discussions between researchers were significant in developing an understanding of the narrative itself (Wertz et al. 2011).

9.6 Results

The narrative explains learning and participation during the life course: learning in communities of practices during childhood and youth, and outsiderness in education and working life. The narrative also contains findings about challenges and how to strengthen learning and participation in education and working life in the future.

9.6.1 Learning in Communities of Practice During Childhood and Youth

Stig enjoyed school and had a good relationship with his teachers. "One trick was to sit at the front of the classroom … It made it easier to follow the lessons". He also had lots of friends and did not identify himself as being visually impaired—that came a lot later in life. "I have always had a positive self-image and never felt that my parents have treated me differently from my siblings. My lack of sight was not a topic ...".

Stig said that during his early school years, he wore very strong reading glasses and could see quite well with them. The biggest concern was around whether he might accidentally break the spectacles because they were expensive, as it would take a long time to procure a new pair. He participated in various sports and was strongly committed. However, he said, laughing, "I was not the first to be selected for the football team—I had no idea where the ball was". This did not bother him at all, as he was able to assert himself in other sports. He also started a sport club together with other boys in his hometown.

At the age of 15 to 16, a blind consultant employed by the regional authority visited his family after he had undergone acute eye surgery on three separate occasions. The blind consultant suggested that he should start adaptation courses at a special school for the blind to prepare for possible blindness in the future. He was sent to boarding school, which was almost 500 km from home, at the age of 17. Eight boys started in a class together and Stig reported that he enjoyed being in this small group together with the others. At boarding school, he learned braille. Stig stated that he has used braille to a small extent during his life, but that he is considering retraining as his residual vision has now disappeared.

At the school for the blind, Stig explained that visually impaired students were required to participate in an aptitude test. It was common at the time to train the visually impaired to become metal workers. It was, however, suggested that he should study at university to become a social worker. Against this background, the choice of profession seemed to be rather random. It transpired that a teacher at the school happened to know a blind person who had become a social worker. "We are talking about coincidences here ..., but it turned out well for me. I enjoyed myself at university, and my later work as a social worker was perceived as meaningful". Stig confided that he always has had a huge interest for mathematics and statistics, but that it was almost impossible for him to read literature that included formulae, tables, and figures because speech synthesis did not support these formats. "Not that I have regretted anything, but had the opportunity been there, I would have probably chosen differently and become a natural scientist ...".

9.6.2 Outsiderness in Education and Working Life

Outsiderness was a recurrent theme in Stig's experiences of participation in various social communities. He talked about existential issues in relation to family life, experience of nature, participation in education and working life, and participation in society.

> One should not forget that vision is the dominant sense for obtaining information from the environment. In many respects one is outside if blind. This is difficult for a sighted person to understand. The emptiness that one might feel as blind ... I haven't dared to take this on yet. Just think what I'm missing out on. The grandchildren's smiles ....

He stated that visual impairment has affected him in a number of ways. He was hindered from participating in following his children's interests, as well as housework, gardening, watching art and movies. He said that he became dependent on his wife regarding practical work and participating in working life. It was a great loss that eventually, he could no longer experience nature. "I would like to be a botanist—to be out in nature much more, but it is difficult".

Stig stated that there was a lack of adapted literature for blind and visually impaired available for both studying and working life. For a long time, he relied on his strong glasses and helped himself by using a magnifying glass. Later on, he got help through speech synthesis on the computer when reading scientific books and papers. He said that his visual impairment probably meant that he tried to adapt early by using the computer as an aid—much earlier than most of his seeing student mates and colleagues did, or indeed, needed to.

Stig reported that he always has been engaged in different organisations related to politic, history, culture, sport, environment, international development, and with questions related to user participation in the health services and in society at large.

He is strongly involved in the National Association of the Visually Impaired in Sweden at regional and national levels. Laughing, he said: “More than 40 memberships in different groups and organisations might be a bit too much—and quite expensive”.

Stig told that he has a high level of social awareness, working for equal conditions, and with issues that deal with sustainability and peace. Moving these issues forward through research has been important for him. After working 10 years as a social worker, he explained that he and his department took the initiative for a development project that resulted in a book. The book had great impact and shed light on various black businesses in society (prostitution, money laundering, and illegal alcohol sales). It rolled on with various projects, and then he was offered a position as a doctoral student in sociology.

Stig’s experience is that no provision has been made for his visual impairment in working life. He became a project manager in various projects and used project money to hire a secretary who took care of the administrative work. “This has come at the expense of not having the money to employ doctoral students within my projects. I have not been given the opportunity to supervise doctoral students as much as I would like. I had to choose between employing administrative help or doctoral students”. The only arrangement he can recall having from the employer was that he was allowed to be accompanied by his wife when attending international conferences.

Stig experienced problems in specially prepared books for the visually impaired in the dissemination of statistics and tables. Statistics and tables are often presented in an unsatisfactory manner. He stated that this makes it difficult to understand the data, as you must get an overview of certain areas of information only found in tables. He described it like this:

> It takes an enormous amount of concentration and energy to get through a table, so I often give up. In other words, it is not just about reading the contents of a table—the reader must ‘understand’ the data and the analyses that the table tries to convey.

Stig considered this as a serious obstacle for visually impaired individuals when trying to participate in science and statistics.

At some conferences, however, he told that he had been offered an on-site companion at the conference. These were usually conferences aimed at research on disabled people. Digital conferences and meetings are extremely difficult to attend. He explained it like this:

> You can’t listen to a presenter, at the same time as the presenter is showing power points, and these are read through speech synthesis, at the same time that there is a moderator, and at the same time that there is a chat function that you should use if you want to ask questions ... Then you have to have a screen reader for the power points and a screen reader for the chat function—as well as to hear the presentation from the lecturer and the moderator. This can be compared to a digital cacophony of voices talking at once ... There are no good solutions for this so far.

He reflected that people with disabilities have always been outside society and unable to participate in various activities. “Nowadays, exclusion is mostly on a symbolic level”. He said that he often experiences outsiderness—also as an academic—especially when attending an international research conference and participating in various social settings. Before the photograph was taken (see Sect. 9.5), the first author found Stig standing alone in a corner. "When you're standing alone as an outsider in a crowd of people—with a glass of wine, I can't mingle like I'm supposed to at a reception at a research conference. I don't recognize anyone".

The photograph was taken after Stig and the first author met. The image expressed experiences of mutual engagement, joy, and cohesion between research colleagues. "This is what acknowledgement and participation in a community of research-practice is about".

Stig has contributed to developing many research fields in both Sweden and internationally. His large production of books and articles documents this. He stated that his research has led to changes in the legislation in Sweden.

9.6.3 *Challenges and Opportunities for Participation in Education and Working Life*

Stig stated that, paradoxically, the IT revolution has given people with visual impairments access to lots of material previously hidden from them. Despite that, this *information explosion* has made it difficult for them to find information quickly. The wide range of information and resources and the difficulty in finding the right information is perceived as problematic. "There are so many clicks and little boxes to deal with …". He continued:

> We can access information online but navigating all these systems is hugely time-consuming. The problem with the screen reader is that it reads everything out. To find a link, for example, you have to listen to the entire text before you get to the information you are looking for. This can take an infinite amount of time.

Stig stated that changes happen so quickly that it is often not worth taking the time to learn how to navigate different systems and webpages. Social media can be difficult to use. Much of the content alludes to images, and Stig said that it is difficult to get good illustrations from visual interpretation of images, not human nor AI interpretation. "Much has happened in the last 10 years, but there is still a long way to go".

Stig reported that lack of individual guidance of various resources and systems is pervasive. There is a need for organisational health literacy to facilitate learning and participation in study and working life. This to enable visually impaired individuals to find, understand, and use information to be active participants in their community of practices. Stig conveyed that there is a need for individual guidance at different levels. This applies to both use and access to digital learning resources and study materials. Follow-up over time and, especially when new solutions are presented, is crucial.

Stig reported that there is a need for adaptation in study literature in books that are read aloud, for example, with regard to page numbers in books and journals. The user needs to be able to navigate the text and also refer to page numbers. Stig told that another problem is that a book which is read aloud has page numbers which do not always correspond exactly with the printed book. In research, it is essential that you can state exactly where you have taken citations from. In e-pub production, page numbers are also often missing, and this is problematic too. It is usually specialist libraries that produce adapted literature. Many books are read by commercial publishers who do not use editable audio files.

Scarce resources in specialist libraries can lead to them using books from commercial publishers rather than producing specially adapted literature for the blind and visually impaired. This can, in turn, lead to a reduced supply of adapted literature which is specifically designed for the end user, rather than books produced for profit.

Various ways of gaining access to adapted literature were mentioned. He could submit a request to a library to have certain literature adapted. He reported that this often takes a long time—up to several months. This impacts his work as a researcher, being able to write a manuscript and meet deadlines. A lack of communication between the library and the users was experienced. Information about if, and when, the book or article would be read was missing. Stig reported that this could be an obstacle to the process of studying and carrying out research. He often contacted the researchers directly and asked for access in Word format. Doing so enables him to then use speech synthesis.

9.7 Discussion

The study provides new and valuable insights into visually impaired individuals' experiences with learning and participation in education and working life. Rich and thick data were obtained. Stories from childhood, youth and education, and working life gave unique findings about learning and participation in different communities of practices for the visually impaired. The interviewees' knowledge and commitment contributed to him being able to convey his own and others' experiences on the topic. A research group with different professional backgrounds was important in the analytical process to create the narrative. This was important for validating the findings (Brinkmann and Kvale 2015). We consider the findings to have transferability to other visually impaired in other countries that have similar educational systems.

The findings show different forms of learning and participation and ways of coping in school and working life. During childhood and youth, good relationships with teachers and fellow pupils were of great significance for positive learning outcomes. Inadequate arrangements in education and working life were described, which resulted in a feeling of outsiderness. Participation in science was particularly challenging, and the choice of profession became limited and random. Individual guidance in the use of digital resources is paramount when attempting to improve full participation in education and working life. There is a need to strengthen specialist competence in the provision of learning resources in order to eliminate barriers to reduce inequalities (SDG 10) and to promote good health and well-being (SDG 3) for the visually impaired.

The interviewee talked about participation in inbound trajectories in childhood and youth. That means that newcomers are joining the community of practice with the prospect of becoming a full participant in a sociocultural practice (Wenger 2004). With the help of strong glasses and good relationships with the teachers and other students, the learning environment was beneficial. His participation in social contexts gave him self-confidence, and he experienced belonging to a community of practice. School was meaningful, and he experienced a mutual engagement in actions. These are, according to Wenger (2004), important elements in becoming a full participant in the community of practice.

The narrative shows that lack of learning resources might prevent visually impaired from choosing education within science. Earlier research has shown that adopted literature in science has not been accessible to blind and visually impaired students (Sahin and Yorek 2009). This may vary between countries, but it is worrying if visually impaired are excluded and discriminated in participation in science. The lack of adapted learning resources and specialist literature for the visually impaired may lead to outbound trajectories towards another community of practice (Wenger 2004).

In education and working life, we found that the environment had a great impact on choices regarding education and working life. Our study shows that the environment may influence what to study and career choices. New relationships and interests may be developed. The interviewee had an interest in science but found another position with respect to the community of practice, changing his identity when becoming a social worker. By becoming a researcher, the interviewee fulfilled his academic ambitions. Wenger (2004) points out that this could be due to various types of trajectories. The study shows coherence through time and connects the past, the present, and the future.

Difficulties in attending digital conferences and meetings were revealed. Attending a digital conference could be experienced as a digital cacophony for the visually impaired as the tools employed were not well coordinated. A study has found that technical systems, such as professional and office systems, are not universally designed (Halbach et al. 2022). Digitalisation opens for increased accessibility if the digitalisation is carried out with a universal design. It seems that a universal design is deficient in both universities and workplaces. Young students who are introduced to new subjects are particularly vulnerable when it comes to insufficient learning resources and a lack of adapted literature. This may lead to outbound trajectories. Participation is a complex process that combines doing, talking, thinking, feeling, and belonging (Wenger 2004). It involves the whole person: it is an active process. It may pose enormous problems when different digital resources are not coordinated.

The narrative demonstrates that the interviewee's participation in education and working life was hindered by obstacles which had major consequences. He experienced outsiderness in a range of different situations. This is in line with earlier research from the United Kingdom (Bishop and Rhind 2011). The interviewee had to make different career choices than those he originally wanted. His participation and "belonging" in social relations also became limited. His academic life was therefore limited, and he had to adjust his academic plans. This came with a personal price. He had to use family and private resources to assist him to be able to participate in academic activities normally expected of a professor.

The narrative highlights discrimination and inequality which can occur in education and working life for visually impaired. Reduced inequalities (SDG 10) and decent work and economic growth (SDG 8) for all are important Sustainability Development Goals. It seems that there is a lack of quality in education (SDG 4) for the visually impaired. Health-literate environment has to be strengthened throughout the life course to obtain good health and well-being (SDG 3). Ensuring environmental support throughout the life course is paramount. Individual and organisational health literacy must be developed on the user's own terms in education and working life.

9.7.1 Strengths and Limitations

The narrative is a construction of events and activities (Flick 2017). The authors have been co-creators in constructing the narrative. Wenger's theory about learning in a community of practices (2004) has been an underpinning framework. The interviewee has been an active participant in the research process and has given suggestions for how to analyse the narratives. He added in-depth knowledge that influenced the design of the interview guide, and he influenced us to choose a user perspective in the study. His last comment on the result section was as follows: "I am impressed by your ability to summarize and to catch important perspectives of my narrative during the interviews" (E-mail correspondence May 27th, 2023). His feedback is a kind of validation of the findings (Brinkmann and Kvale 2015).

The researchers have different academic positions such as social science, health science, sociology, and language and linguistic with special competence in the preparation of literature and learning resources for the visually impaired. These different competences were important in the analyses of the different data sources as well as the presentation of the results.

In this study, we chose to interview one, sole, interviewee. The data were rich and thick (Flick 2017) throughout their lifespan. The narratives can be understood as a historical and biographical narrative; however, we created a narrative about learning and participating in education and working life. The interviewee, of course, has his own historical perspective; he is still an internationally recommended researcher at Lund University.

It may be seen as a weakness that we only have one interviewee. In this study, we consider it as a strength because it presented an opportunity to gain in-depth knowledge about learning and participation. The interviewee's age, knowledge, experience, and commitment provided unique data from a life course perspective. In the discussion section, we compare the interviewee's narrative with earlier research in the field. This was the way in which we validated our findings.

9.8 Conclusion and Relevance to Clinical Practice

The study provides new insights into the visually impaired people's experiences of learning and participation in education and working life. It appears that the visually impaired are often discriminated against, and experience inequalities in the important spheres of education and working life. Visually impaired individuals do not have access to the adapted resources which they need to be fully integrated in society and to live full, and fulfilling, lives.

Implications for Practice

- Coping and participation in school and working life is important for good health and well-being.
- It is crucial to improve participation and increased access to learning resources for the visually impaired.
- Visually impaired individuals' health literacy needs to be developed at individual and organisational levels on their own terms.
- Access to personal guidance is vital for coping with rapid development in digitalisation and preventing outsiderness.
- There is a need to strengthen expertise in special libraries in adapting literature for education and research.
- Universal design in digital resources globally is paramount.
- Global partnerships are important in adapting learning resources for the visually impaired in an effective and sustainable way.

References

Accessible Books Consortium (ABC) (2023) Global book services. https://www.accessiblebooksconsortium.org/en/web/abc/globalbooks. Accessed 21 May 2023

Bishop D, Rhind DJA (2011) Barriers and enablers for visually impaired students at a UK higher education institution. Br J Vis Impair 29:3. https://doi.org/10.1177/0264619611415329

Brinkmann S, Kvale S (2015) InterViews: learning the craft of qualitative research interviewing, 3rd edn. Sage, Thousand Oaks

Brunes A, Hansen B, Heir T (2019) Loneliness among adults with visual impairment: prevalence, associated factors, and relationship to life satisfaction. Health Qual Life Outcomes 17(1). https://doi.org/10.1186/s12955-019-1096-y

Centers for Disease Control and Prevention, CDC (2020) What is health literacy. Available at: https://www.cdc.gov/healthliteracy/learn/index.html

Chase SE (2018) Narrative inquiry toward theoretical and methodological maturity. In: Denzin NK, Lincoln YS (eds) The Sage handbook of qualitative research, 5th edn. Sage, Los Angeles

Creswell JW, Creswell JD (2018) Research design: qualitative, quantitative and mixed methods approaches, 5th edn. SAGE Publications Inc., Los Angeles

Demmin DL, Silverstein SM (2020) Visual impairment and mental health: unmet needs and treatment options. Clin Ophthalmol 14:4229–4251

Dhital A, Pey T, Stanford MR (2010) Visual loss and falls: a review. Eye 24(9):1437–1446. https://doi.org/10.1038/eye.2010.60

Flick U (2017) An introduction to qualitative research, 6th edn. Sage Publication Ltd., London

French S (2017) Visual impairment and work. Experiences of visually impaired people. Routledge, London

Ganz A, Barnoy D, Amedi A (2020) The impact of assistive technology on the employment of people with visual impairments: a systematic review. J Visual Impair Blin 114(6):619–635

Gordois A, Cutler H, Pezzullo L et al (2012) An estimation of the worldwide economic and health burden of visual impairment. Glob Public Health 7(5):465–481. https://doi.org/10.1080/17441692.2011.634815

Halbach T, Fyhn T, Fuglerud KS, Kjæret K, Olsen TA (2022) Kanskje du kunne bli maler?—Fem personer med nedsatt syn forteller om sine erfaringer som arbeidssøkere og arbeidstakere [Maybe you could become a painter?—Five people with reduced vision talk about their experiences as job seekers and employees]. Norges Blindeforbund, Oslo

Holloway I, Freshwater D (2007) Narrative research in nursing. Blackwell, Oxford

Khorrami-Nejad M, Sarabandi A, Akbari M-R, Askarizadeh F (2016) The impact of visual impairment on quality of life. Med Hypothesis Discov Innov Ophthalmol 5(3):96–103

Kylberg M, Haak M, Iwarsson S (2018) Research with and about user participation: potentials and challenges. Aging Clin Exp Res 30:105–108. https://doi.org/10.1007/s40520-017-0750-7

Marrakesh Treaty (2013) National library service marrakesh treaty implementation. https://www.loc.gov/nls/about/organization/laws-regulations/marrakesh-treaty/. Accessed 21 May 2023

Patton MQ (2015) Qualitative research & evaluation methods: integrating theory and practice, 4th edn. SAGE Publications, Los Angeles

Proba Research (2019) Universell utforming av IKT med vekt på læremidler i UH-sektoren [Universal design of ICT with an emphasis on teaching aids in the university sector]

Sahin M, Yorek N (2009) Teaching science to visually impaired students: a small-scale qualitative study. US-China Educ Rev 6(53):19–26

Shippee ND, Domecq Garces JP, Prutsky Lopez GJ et al (2013) Patient and service user engagement in research: a systematic review and synthesized framework. Health Expect 18:1151–1166

Swedish Council for Higher Education (2015) [Universitets- och högskolerådet]. Eurostudent V: A brief insight into the situation for students with disabilities [Eurostudent V: En kort inblick i situationen för studenter med funktionsnedsättning]. https://www.uhr.se/globalassets/_uhr.se/lika-mojligheter/eurostudent/eurostudentv-funk-150624.pdf. Accessed 12 Dec 2023

Swedish Radio—P4 Halland (2012, December 3) Funktionsnedsatta har en mörk historia [The disabled have a dark history]. https://sverigesradio.se/artikel/5367146. Accessed 12 Mar 2023

The Norwegian Association of the Blind (2023) [Norges Blindeforbund]. Synstap og psykisk helse [Vision loss and mental health]. ISBN 978-82-8122-168-0

The Norwegian Library of Talking Books and Braille (2017) [Norsk lyd- og blindeskriftbibliotek, NLB] Bedre tilgang til studielitteratur [Better access to study literature]. Norway, Oslo

The Swedish Code of Statutes (2005) [Svensk forfattningssamling, SFS] Lag (2003:460) om etikprövning av forskning som avser människor [Law on ethical review of research involving humans]. http://www.riksdagen.se/sv/Dokument-Lagar/Lagar/Svenskforfattningssamling/Lag-2003460-om-etikprovning_sfs-2003-460/. Accessed 8 July 2023

Wenger E (2004) Community of practice—learning, meaning and identity. Cambridge University Press, Cambridge

Wenger E (2011) Communities of practice—a brief introduction, page 1. https://scholarsbank.uoregon.edu/xmlui/handle/1794/11736. Accessed 6 July 2023

Wertz FJ, McSpadden E, Charmaz K et al (2011) Five ways of doing qualitative analysis: phenomenological psychology, grounded theory, discourse analysis, narrative research and intuitive inquiry. Guilford Publication, New York

World Medical Association (2013) World Medical Association Declaration of Helsinki ethical principles for medical research involving human subjects. Available https://www.wma.net/policies-post/wma-declaration-of-helsinki-ethical-principles-for-medical-research-involving-human-subjects/

Chapter 10
Empowering Agency: Enhancing Health Literacy Among Migrant Women Through Health Parties: A Case Study

Marianne Hedlund, Yan Zhao, and Trude Karine Olaug Gjernes

Abstract This chapter explores how agency involvement through Health Parties can generate and promote learning agencies for migrant women to enforce health literacy. The Norwegian healthcare system struggles to provide sufficient responses to the needs of current and potential patients of the migrant population, particularly migrant women. A lack of cultural sensitivity and a more bottom-up approach is needed. Inspired by *Tupperware Parties*, this chapter explores the model of Health Parties, initiated by the female network of migrant women, called *Kvinnenettverket Noor* in Norwegian. A Health Party is based on a model where a host invites female friends, family, and acquaintances to a party to share information and learn about a relevant health issue by creating an appropriate space for discussion among experts and participants. This model can be employed when working to fulfil the United Nations Sustainable Development Goals concerning health and equity for migrant women. An explorative qualitative community-based participatory study design was employed. Data were collected by analysing participant observations and semi-structured face-to-face interviews in seven arranged Health Parties from September 2015 to March 2016. Health Parties generate learning agencies by providing space for active participation for migrant women. The healthcare system, which is based on Norwegian norms and culture, created cultural alienation and barriers that migrant women need space and knowledge to overcome. The results show the need for a public healthcare system and its professionals to be more sensitive and better adjusted to cultural diversity. They also provide insights into how migrant women gain agency about health issues by attending a Health Party. New ways of communication are required and found in the model of Health Parties for addressing health literacy among migrant women.

The original version of the chapter has been revised. A correction to this chapter can be found at https://doi.org/10.1007/978-3-031-61810-9_13

M. Hedlund (✉)
Department of Social Work, Norwegian University of Science and Technology (NTNU), Trondheim, Norway
e-mail: marianne.hedlund@ntnu.no

Y. Zhao · T. K. O. Gjernes
Faculty of Social Sciences, Nord University, Bodø, Norway

T. Hole et al. (eds.), *Towards Sustainable Good Health and Well-being*,
https://doi.org/10.1007/978-3-031-61810-9_10

Keywords Migrant women · Health parties · Cultural diversity · Ethnicity · Collective learning

10.1 Introduction

In this chapter, we address agency involvement among migrant women and discuss how a model of a Health Party contributed to generating and promoting learning agencies for migrant women. Norway's public healthcare system is based on public financing, universal health coverage, and culturally socialised "taken-for-granted knowledge" of accessing and using the health system. Despite the existence of an indigenous population, the Sami, and national minorities, Norway has traditionally been perceived to be a homogeneous society with *one* culture where information about the Public Health care system was passed on to the same ethnic population and between generations. However, with global mass immigration, there are significant populations of immigrants and their descendants from various countries. The Norwegian government promotes equality and diversity, and the country has policies to support multiculturalism and integration. Since 2018, there has been a rapid rise in the number of international migrants, accounting for more than 10% of the European and 16% of the Norwegian population (Diaz and Kumar 2018). As Norway undergoes a significant demographic change with increasing heterogeneity, the country is also experiencing an increase in social inequality in health, including risks such as poor living conditions accompanied by poor health outcomes among groups of immigrants (Abebe et al. 2017; Goldblatt et al. 2023; Statistics Norway 2023). Immigrants and Norwegian-born individuals with immigrant parents are a complex group with different reasons for immigration, ethnic, and socio-economic backgrounds: this may impact risk factors for disease, the use of health services, and expectations and demands on and for healthcare services. There are differences in their levels of health literacy. Recent and previous migrant populations, including refugees, may not be familiar with how the Norwegian healthcare system is organised and may experience encounters with the healthcare system as discriminatory, or lacking cultural sensitivity. There can be various reasons behind this challenge, including the lack of knowledge about cultural sensitivity for minorities to access welfare and healthcare services in Norway (Moe and Hedlund 2019; Hedlund and Moe 2010). Most European countries' policies have strived towards equitable welfare and health services to citizens regardless of ethnicity, religion, region, country of origin, and other characteristics. Yet the literature describes challenges in providing healthcare for multicultural populations by doctors and other healthcare professionals (Varvin and Aasland 2009; Debesay et al. 2014). Making healthcare responsive to patients' and locals' needs remains a work in progress. This may be particularly apparent in the lack of sensitivity to the healthcare needs of migrant women. Biological differences and sociocultural variations related to gender must also be considered when dealing with a diverse patient and client group. Recent health policy reforms have stressed the need for better patient and public involvement (Kasper et al. 2022). By 2011, it was claimed that existing involvement mechanisms in Norway were dominated by suggestions from health professionals and their interests (Solbjør and Steinsbekk 2011). Later, researchers claimed that in Scandinavia, few approaches to health research highlight the needs and priorities of migrants, particularly migrant women (Bradby et al. 2015). An approach highlighting the needs and priorities of migrant women will be essential because it can inform the public healthcare system about how best to access these women's well-being and good health. By so doing, it will also contribute to several of the Sustainable Development Goals (SDGs) by the United Nations, such as SDG 3: Good health and well-being, SDG 5: Gender equality, and SDG 10: Reduced inequalities. This chapter provides a concrete case of such an approach. Called a *Health Party*, inspired by *Tupperware Parties*, a host invites female friends, family, and acquaintances to a party, where the goal, besides being a social event, is to share information about a health-related topic and create a space for discussion.

10.2 Health Literacy and Migrant Women in Norway

In the Norwegian context, health literacy refers to a person's ability to find, understand, assess, and apply health information in a way that enables this person to make knowledge-based decisions related to health (Norwegian Health Directorate 2021). For Norwegian health authorities, health literacy means having competence when making decisions about lifestyle choices, disease prevention measures, disease self-management, and use of health and care services. Health literacy will relate to individual and system-oriented efforts. In 2021, a survey was carried out in Norway about health literacy from five selected immigrant groups following citizenship and/or place of birth: Pakistan, Poland, Somalia, Turkey, or Vietnam, called the HLS19, part 2 (Le et al. 2021). This survey showed that one out of three had low levels of general health literacy in these migrant populations and that migrant persons who score low on health literacy might lack critical skills for meeting expectations in the health system in general and in individual health services. The survey did not focus on migrant women or sex-gender issues. On a general basis, the survey showed that migrants from these countries found it difficult to navigate the healthcare system and challenging to find information about how to handle mental health problems.

Migrants from non-Western backgrounds in Norway have, very generally, poorer health outcomes compared with the native population on some measures, and women are even more affected than men, according to research (Forland 2009; Blom 2011). Individually, many migrants are more likely to be exposed to certain illnesses and health problems such as diabetes, HIV, hepatitis B, tuberculosis, lack of vitamin D, and mental health problems (Spilker et al. 2009). Migrants may face health risks and challenges related to socio-economic, cultural, religious, and gender backgrounds. Their interactions with health care providers and welfare services can be shaped by what migrant women consider to be the political, legal, and gender regimes and accepted norms in their host country. Choices and actions related to health and sickness will influence their experience accessing and using health services (Attanapola 2013; Diaz and Kumar 2018). Consequently, the way in which migrant women relate to health literacy and make informed choices about the use of health care is not entirely a learning process predetermined by their original cultural background. Thus, migrant women must acquire new strategies for interacting with new and unfamiliar healthcare systems.

Other research demonstrates that culture and migration are two different determinants of health (Thurston and Vissandjée 2005) and that the migration experience is often overlooked, or confused with, culture. Similarly, the extent to which ethnicity and culture, including cultural and religious practices, influence health status and outcomes is heavily contested (Abebe 2010; Balaam et al. 2013; Viken et al. 2015; Kale et al. 2018). Cultural differences, for example, holding a different explanatory model of health and illness, can impact the relationship between health professionals and patients/service users and influence the delivery of services (Avis et al. 2008). It is also reasonable to think that these differences in ethnic and cultural background can influence migrant women's health literacy and thus impact the use of health services and health outcomes. Migration is a complex and dynamic process that can alter and exaggerate health inequalities linked to individual, social, environmental, and health-related factors (Abebe 2010). The health of migrants and their use of health services has recently received more attention in European countries (Debesay et al. 2014; Indseth et al. 2021). Studies in Norway and other Western countries identify significant variations in health status between and even within ethnic groups and a strong association between ethnicity and health outcomes (Kumar et al. 2004; Jenum et al. 2005; Kinnunen et al. 2019; Stalheim et al. 2023).

During the pandemic, we learned that migrant groups might be more vulnerable, both individually and on a collective level, in terms of their ability to understand public health information (Indseth et al. 2021; Hussaini and Ezzati 2022). Previous studies in Norway also document a significant disparity between some immigrant women's own culture and that of the host society regarding gender expectations; immigrant women often feel powerless and marginalised (Attanapola 2013). However, to be effective in the communication about health issues between health and welfare providers, who usually belong to the majority population, the migrant population requires an understanding and engagement in cultural issues rather than simply preparing information materials in other languages and using interpreters (Ask and Berg 2011; Diaz and Kumar 2018; Zhao et al. 2021). Migrants' and particularly migrant women's perspectives and priorities must also be given attention to give them equal access to health care (Bradby et al. 2015; Lebano et al. 2020).

10.3 Health Party as Learning Agency

Learning about using health information and interacting with health and welfare services can be addressed as shaping agencies. That is a process where actors learn how to break down complexity into manageable steps that can be understood and used when interacting with health care services. The agency is then understood as a process for how migrant women engage and enact the social structure of a Public Health care system. The concept of agency, as understood by Giddens (1984), emphasises practical consciousness and how persons relate to social actions in a system. According to Giddens, there will always be a relationship between learning about agency in a duality of specific structures. Individuals' ability to be reflective will produce and reproduce the knowledge they need in their social life. This requires that migrant women actively participate in the learning process, putting themselves at the centre of the learning, while relating their life situations and experiences to the information being disseminated. Through this active participatory learning, they also learn to be agents in the health care system, having acquired knowledge about when and where to seek help and information and how the system can benefit them.

A Health Party is a bottom-up community programme developed by *Kvinnenettverket Noor* (hereafter NOOR), a women's organization initiated by migrant women. This programme aims to influence how migrant women focus on, learn about, and discuss health issues as well as how they interact with health care (Zhao et al. 2021). This implies that Health Parties could inspire migrant women to reflect and interact with healthcare systems. The term "Health Party" is not used here as a widely recognised term in science. It refers to a bottom-up initiative and method where social gatherings or events promote health and well-being. Just like a Tupperware party, where individuals gather to socialise and purchase Tupperware products, a Health Party may involve women coming together to learn about and discuss various health topics, participate in health-related activities, and are possibly willing to "purchase" or consume health information or services (Zhao et al. 2021). A Health Party as a social gathering aims to create a supportive and empowering environment for migrant women to address their needs and concerns regarding interactions with doctors or other health and welfare service providers. A Health Party is often organised by community organisations, or individual community members interested in promoting health and wellness for their communities. The specific activities and topics covered during a Health Party may vary depending on the organisers' and participants' needs and interests. Health parties combine educational presentations of health-related topics with social activities, such as informal group discussions, cooking, sharing a meal, yoga, or mindfulness practice. These events may also provide an opportunity for migrant women to access healthcare resources, understand information, and discuss health worries and health conditions with professionals or local health service providers and programmes. By participating in a Health Party, a health professional gets access to migrant women's health and information needs and their perspectives and cultural premises for utilising health care services.

By creating a relaxed and social atmosphere, a Health Party can help migrant women overcome cultural and language barriers, promote health equity, and empower them to take charge of their well-being. All these facilitate the shaping of the learning agency and ensure migrant women's active participation in learning. The Health Party can teach migrant women to reflect more on their interactions with healthcare professionals. Migrant women get access to priorities regarding shared decision-making and user involvement in interactions with healthcare professionals. Compared to traditional patient involvement approaches that often reinforce existing societal hierarchies and adopt a top-down expert-driven health communication model, a Health Party will represent a bottom-up, user-driven approach (Zhao et al. 2021; Mehrara et al. 2022). Health Parties represent an integrated, coherent patient and user pathway that may teach migrant women how to improve user skills and utilise health information. This chapter examines the role of Health Parties in fostering agency among migrant women, specifically focusing on their impact on learning and promoting health literacy.

10.4 Research Design and Methods

10.4.1 Design

The current study is inspired by the approach of "community-based participatory research" (CBPR) (Hacker 2017). This design conducts research focusing on collaboration between a partner that initiates a project, community members, and other stakeholders (Hacker 2017). In the case of Health Parties, data is collected from the main stakeholders, the hosts, and the participants. The CBPR approach recognises the significance of securing participation by social groups in the research processes (Cargo and Mercer 2008; Alcalde-Rabanal et al. 2018). CBRP promotes a democratic and inclusive approach to research, fostering collaboration and empowering communities or social groups to participate actively in the entire research process (Isaacs et al. 2020).

10.4.2 Methods

The study is based on data collected from NOOR's Health Party project through participant observations and semi-structured interviews. Other results from this project are published elsewhere (Zhao 2017; Zhao et al. 2021). The data for results presented here was collected by a researcher with a migrant background during Autumn 2015 and Spring 2016. She participated in seven Health Parties, four of which took place in private homes; the other three took place in borrowed meeting rooms. The topics discussed at the different Health Parties varied and covered topics such as diabetes and diet, asthma and allergies, thyroid disorders, mental health and coping with stress, reproductive health, menopause, and an HPV screening programme. Detailed notes were recorded after each of the Health Parties, focusing on the contents and forms of interactions carried out and the informal conversations the researcher had with participants and the resource persons during the Health Parties. The five hosts who arranged these seven Health Parties and, one resource person, a gynaecologist who has a migrant background and attended several Health Parties were interviewed about their experiences at Health Parties as well as their reflections.

10.4.3 Participants

The participants at the Health Parties belong to different migrant communities in the same Norwegian county. They originally came from Asian, African, and Latin American countries. The participants in the interviews were hosts at the Health Parties. These hosts were often key figures in local migrant communities. One of the hosts was a Norwegian social worker, a lead figure in a local project promoting the work and social participation of migrant women in particular. One interviewee attended several Health Parties as a resource person/health professional. Observations were of both participants and their interactions at seven Health Parties. The number of participants in the studied Health Parties varied: the most minor Health Party had five participants while the largest had 12. The age of the participants varied from 17 years old to mid-50s. Their time of residence in Norway varied from several months up to 20 years, which means that their proficiency in the Norwegian language also varied. In most Health Parties, participants with better proficiency in Norwegian helped those relatively new in Norway with translation when needed. A translator was engaged only in one Health Party where participants used different mother tongues, and one participant was a newly arrived migrant.

10.4.4 Ethics

The Norwegian Data Protection Service (NSD: Project No. 46809) granted ethical approval to study the Health Parties. Anonymity and digression were secured as a condition of data access. Informed consent was provided by all participants and interviewees at seven Health Parties. No participant objected to the researcher's access to the Health Party. The participants and interviewees were informed of their rights to withdraw from the research process at any time and assured that any data related to them would be deleted. Also, participants were informed that the data collection contained information about the composition among the participants, relationships, and interactions with each other and communication and interaction between the resource person(s) in addition to the atmosphere, the role of the host, and the role of the active and passive participants. The researcher also emphasised external conditions that influenced the execution of the Health Party, such as seating arrangements, projector/IT equipment, catering, and brochures provided.

10.4.5 *Analysis*

The research interviews were transcribed verbatim, including the field notes from the researcher's observations, and then all data were analysed. Included in the data analysis was information about how and by whom the Health Party was organised, the topic of each Health Party, and more detailed information on how the participants interacted with each other; to what degree did the experts give the information that was understood; and to what degree did the migrant woman ask questions, share their experiences, and find the topics relevant and useful.

A thematic analysis was undertaken (Braun and Clarke 2006). The data material was coded, read several times, and discussed among the research team (authors of this chapter). Ideas about the overall research question emerged and were discussed. Patterns were identified and re-coded. There were codes about access to health information, collaboration, participatory voice, individual and collective learning, language problems, experiences from interaction with the resource person/professional, use of technology, and cultural diversity. These were during a rigorous process of discussion and review of data merged into the two main themes: (1) *Key ability to seek health information* and (2) *cultural sensitivity in identifying health issues*. We describe and discuss these two themes in the coming sections, demonstrating how they contribute to answering the research question on how the Health Party contributes to generating and promoting learning agencies for migrant women.

10.5 Results

10.5.1 *Key to Seeking and Understanding Health Information*

The results show that participating in Health Parties equipped migrant women with fundamental abilities about how they should seek and receive healthcare information. Those who hosted Health Parties were mostly migrant women themselves. This made the hosts emphasise the importance of accessing knowledge and how it was even more critical to be able to address questions together with others at the Health Party and with the healthcare professional in attendance. One expressed it like this:

> Yes, I have been to other information meetings, not really as a receiver of information, but as an interpreter for such meetings. These meetings concern children and schools, and I was there as an interpreter. Yes. That's how you received the information. If we compare them to Health Parties, then maybe Health Parties are more detailed, ... with aids, projector, and

> other things. So maybe it's better because there are so many... [facilitations]. You can also understand and speak or ask questions. But when you are in a large group, you lose some information, or when you are interpreting, because everyone is talking. It was a mixed group. And it wasn't just me who was the interpreter. There were also Russian, Somali, and other languages. (Informant A)

The informant compared Health Parties with other information meetings she participated in as a migrant and language interpreter. According to her, what makes Health Parties different is that it provides more space for learning, in the informant's own words, room to "understand", to "speak" with other participants, and to "ask" questions, which is related to size (a much smaller group) and the informal setting. She also talked about facilities, including the projector. Several participants spoke about the positive effects of using PowerPoint slides, which make it easier to follow the information given and more manageable to ask questions because, for many participants, spoken Norwegian, with different dialects, is more complex than written Norwegian. Therefore, Health Parties facilitate an arena-generating learning agency by providing space for learning, and technology like a projector, in addition to an informal setting, invites active participation and discussion.

The data analysis revealed that the experience of participation at a Health Party lowered the barrier to asking questions about the topic being addressed, even if the information was given in Norwegian. There was a 15-min break at one Health Party after the resource person finished the presentation. Several of the participants were new arrivals in Norway and were not so familiar with the Norwegian language. They started asking each other: "How much have you understood?" They told the researcher that this is not only a question of understanding the information given but also of learning from listening to "the real Norwegian," in other words, to practice how you communicate in Norwegian outside a classroom and in "real situations". They said it might be about what they did and did not understand. Shortly after the break, when the resource person started talking again, she was asked whether she could use *Bokmål* instead of her dialect, which some participants perceived as challenging to understand. *Bokmål* is one of the official Norwegian languages and a more literary language than many Norwegian dialects (except Oslo and its close surroundings). When speaking the (more formal) language of *Bokmål,* it became more accessible for the participants to understand the information given. Newly arrived migrants unfamiliar with the dialect in their area, they expressed the importance of getting to know people and Norwegian society in general. They stated that this was a motivation for attending a Health Party. Meanwhile, they expressed the need to *know more about the Norwegian system, for example, what is available/accessible and what kind of rights you have as a patient.*

These diverse and interrelated needs shaped the migrants' motivation to attend a Health Party. The analysis showed how this motivation could be interpreted as a prerequisite for willingness to learn. The participants positioned themselves as real active learning subjects, not merely passively receiving information. Several hosts underlined this aspect, which was confirmed in the analysed observations. Hosts expressed that migrant women were more active and curious at the Health Party than their experiences with women attending other settings and "information meetings". Some migrant women were curious about what a Health Party was, and during the Health Party, they expressed more awareness of their needs for information and well-being. By discussing issues and asking questions, migrant women participating in a Health Party develop an agency in a supportive environment. The resources activated through participation in a Health Party provided new insights and guidance that migrant women could use in their interactions with healthcare services. Participation in a Health Party taught migrant women the importance of creating a supportive and inclusive environment where cultural and language barriers could be overcome, promoting health equity, and encouraging them to take an active role in their well-being. This indicates that the Health Party became a learning arena for active participation, which gave migrant women valuable experience in their ability to seek health information and learn.

10.5.2 *Cultural Familiarity and Sensitivity in Collective Learning*

When planning a Health Party, the host decides the topic. However, sometimes new health issues or topics were also identified during a Health Party. For example, one host who was a nurse herself first arranged a Health Party about the topic of HPV infection and cervical cancer because she had read about migrant women being under-represented in their participation in the screening programme in Norway. During this Health Party and particularly during informal discussions, the new topic of menopause came up. The participants then decided collectively that they wanted another Health Party focusing on menopause, and they immediately invited the same resource person, a gynaecologist, to come to the new Health Party.

The host needed to discuss relevant health issues related to the chosen topic with her guests and the resource person. Resource persons often expressed a need to have at least some information about the guests before a Health Party because they consider this information could help them prepare for the presentation. Some hosts said they discussed what might interest the participants when communicating with a resource person. In this way, the host, who knew the potential participants, was essential in identifying relevant health issues to discuss. This also ensured that the resource person would talk in a supportive way and be sensitive to cultural differences. From the observed data, the Health Party created a supportive and inclusive environment where cultural and language barriers were overcome. Because the participants knew each other well, asking and participating in conversations was easier. They also helped each other to translate questions. The host and those who had stayed in Norway longer also helped explain the information. This highlights the positive effects of promoting learning agency through collective learning, which has a community-oriented empowerment approach (Ansari et al. 2012).

This meant that the resource persons were required to visit the Health Party outside of their office hours and to talk about health issues in a "non-clinic setting", that is, a setting where they were not consulted to assist, treat, or address a personal sickness or health issue, but to share, not only their pieces of knowledge but sometimes also life experiences. The resource person needed to promote health equity and diminish distance to the participants to encourage them to speak about their health and well-being. A gynaecologist, an Arab migrant, attended as a resource person at several health parties. She used her background and experiences when addressing health issues. She could tell, based on her cultural background and experience as a migrant, what would be strange or difficult to talk about. Meanwhile, as a professional working in the Norwegian healthcare system, she also knew what information was necessary for the migrant women to know. Some participants described her as very "pleasant" to talk with. Here is a quote illustrating how cultural background and sensitivity could lower barriers to speaking about and identifying health issues:

> Host: …… Yes, many of us are shy. So, it is good to have the security that they can ask.
>
> Interviewer: Yes, I saw a lot of people asking the resource person questions.
> Host: XX (name of the expert) is very pleasant. I also think they [the participants] see her as part of us, right? She also has an ethnic minority background, and you feel a kind of togetherness when she talks -don't you? When she talked about the gynecologic test which is part of [name of the Norwegian national screening program], she emphasized that it is for all Norwegian women, including us. When we moved to Norway, we were included in statistics.
>
> Interviewer: So, do you think that the fact that XX has a migrant background contributed to more questions from the participants?
>
> Host: Yes, also, because the topic is gynecologist examination and HPV, they [the participants] want a female doctor. So, in a way, XX got through to this group. Because many want a female doctor. When it's a female doctor, they're not so shy.

This means that the resource person worked to create a sense of familiarity and cultural understanding when addressing health issues. This made the participants identify with the resource person, creating a sense of "community" between the health expert and the participants at the Health Party. Participants overcame the "shyness" and created a safe atmosphere to ask, speak, and learn. The experience of talking about health issues at the Health Party could be an eye-opener for migrant women to overcome shyness and talk about other health issues of general concern. As one host who arranged several Health Parties expressed, "*There is more 'health' and less 'party' when a Health Party is arranged. People got more aware of their health in general*". In this way, the Health Parties create a bridge over "troubled waters" about health issues complex to discuss in public due to shyness or cultural differences. As one host who herself worked in the health care system said:

> I thought afterwards that we could have more parties, more [health] topics, because there is a lot of information that has not reached people, especially in our group. I have the impression that many people do not understand the symptoms they may have, for example, diabetes, metabolism, and menopause; there is so much you could get information about. It is pretty useful. Health Parties are a reasonable proposition. We could also talk about these topics after you [the resource people and the researcher] left, right? Because we don't usually talk about these topics. We are a little too shy to talk to the doctor about anything. Because we feel that, yes, many of us are shy. So, it is good to experience security so that they can ask. (informant E)

The results show that when migrant women discuss at the Health Party with a resource person working as a health specialist who was migrant, it creates an atmosphere of trust. This contributes to migrant women exploring and asking questions about disease risk and how to improve health and well-being. This experience made migrant women overcome their shyness about talking to professionals about sensitive or private topics and made them communicate confidently. The migrant women expressed relief that the party did not follow a strict timeline for consultancy and discussion so they could reflect and develop at their own pace. If wanted, the participants could stay longer, and they often continued the discussion and even shared the information further with other friends who did not come to the Health Party. When several participants found the topic interesting, it created a new awareness about addressing health issues in interactions with professionals and what was most relevant to discuss.

10.6 Discussion

The analysis of the first theme (key ability to seek and understand health information) shows that the Health Party provides a platform for migrant women to learn about health issues and how to take action. As per Giddens' (1984) theory on agency, the Health Party is an effective platform for empowering migrant women with knowledge and skills related to health issues, enabling them to take charge of their well-being. In line with Abebe (2010) and Abebe et al. (2017), this study confirms that migrant women can represent a complex group with different backgrounds. They may share a common experience of an unfamiliar healthcare system and what influences their choices and interactions (Thurston and Vissandjée 2005). Health Parties provide a platform for sharing knowledge and actively seeking and interpreting health information together in an informal setting. This setting lowers the barrier of language issues or other challenges to understanding the information given. Thus, in the setting of a Health Party, migrant women understand more and become less vulnerable in their ability to understand the health information provided (Debesay et al. 2014). The experiences and knowledge gained through Health Parties empower migrant women with the skills to navigate information that may otherwise hinder their access to healthcare services and impede this system's ability to answer their questions (Bradby et al. 2015; Lebano et al. 2020). Health Parties, therefore, create a "safe space" for learning how to use health information and interacting with health and welfare services.

Discussion of the second theme (cultural familiarity and sensitivity in collective learnings) shows that migrant women at the Health Party overcame challenges for doctors to provide healthcare for multicultural populations (Debesay et al. 2014; Varvin and Aasland 2009). This happened when a doctor was open about their migrant experiences and were sensitive to multicultural diversity when addressing health issues. Thus, essential skills to meet expectations of migrant women or sex-gendered issues in health care means involving health professionals with awareness to be culturally sensitive (Hedlund and Moe 2010) and allowing for solid patient involvement in the consultation (Kasper et al. 2022). We found that the Health Party was a platform for building trust between health professionals and healthcare users. It created a space for learning to have safe discussions about delicate issues that some migrant women consider "private" in a group setting. Experiences from the Health Party could unease the way migrant women navigate the healthcare system and how they understand public health information (Zhao et al. 2021; Hussaini and Ezzati 2022). Learning agency through the platform of a Health Party shows how migrant women's awareness and knowledge about health issues improved and made them search for pathways which were helpful for them to be comfortable and cope with interactions with health professionals. All these positive results are essential aspects of health literacy, particularly as to an individual's ability to seek and understand facts and information, as well as the development of communicative and interactive skills (Nutbeam 2000).

10.7 Conclusion

This chapter offers insights into how Health Parties foster health literacy and learning agencies among migrant women. As the introduction highlights, the migrant population, especially migrant women, requires increased competency to engage with the Norwegian healthcare system.

Throughout the chapter, we demonstrate that learning agency, cultivated through participation in Health Parties, provides a space for active involvement. Migrant women, through these events, not only gain a better understanding of health issues but also learn to ask questions, reflect, and address health concerns collaboratively with professionals. This approach allows them to develop agencies tailored to their specific needs for health information and practice Norwegian language skills in real-life situations, thereby promoting health literacy on an individual level. The analysis underscores the significance of technical facilitation and cultural sensitivity in identifying health issues, emphasising the positive effects of collective learning. These aspects create a safe, supportive, and trustful atmosphere, reducing barriers to participation in health communication. Migrant women, as a result, develop increased awareness and knowledge about health issues, fostering confidence in navigating the Norwegian public health care system and overcoming potential barriers. This, in turn, contributes to learning agencies at both the individual and collective levels of health literacy.

Health Parties for migrant women as a bottom-up community health programme can thus have positive outcomes as to the UN's Sustainable Development Goal (SDG) 3, (Good health and well-being). Given the topics that were usually taken up in the health parties, it particularly contributes to 3.7 Sexual and reproductive health, 3.1 Maternal morbidity, and 3.2 Neonatal and child morbidity. Since the ability to access the Norwegian health systems was a major focus when these health issues were discussed at the Health Parties, it also contributes to 3.8 Universal health coverage under SDG 3. Meanwhile, the findings underscore the need for a culturally sensitive public health system in Norway that accommodates diversity, moving away from a system centred on Norwegian (majority) culture and customs. Such an approach can improve health literacy at both individual and systemic levels.

10.8 Implications

The study's implications for Health Parties suggest that the development of these platforms may enhance health literacy for migrant women. It is crucial for Norwegian health authorities to collaborate with migrant communities, employing bottom-up strategies to disseminate health information and address health-related issues. The Health Parties model could be expanded more extensively, providing more migrant women with opportunities to access information and prioritise health issues daily. This expanded approach could contribute to more significant equity in healthcare access and health information seeking for migrant women. It will also teach healthcare systems competence to approach migrant women with more cultural sensitivity.

References

Abebe DS (2010) Public health challenges of immigrants in Norway: a research review. Report, Norwegian Center for Minority Health Research, Oslo

Abebe DS, Lien L, Elstad JI (2017) Immigrants' utilization of specialist mental healthcare according to age, country of origin, and migration history: a nation-wide register study in Norway. Soc Psychiatry Psychiatr Epidemiol 52:679–687

Alcalde-Rabanal JE, Becerril-Montekio VM, Langlois EV (2018) Evaluation of communities of practice performance developing implementation research to enhance maternal health decision-making in Mexico and Nicaragua. Implement Sci 13:41–41

Ansari S, Munir K, Gregg T (2012) Impact at the 'Bottom of the Pyramid': the role of social capital in capability development and community empowerment. J Manag Stud 49:813–842

Ask TA, Berg B (2011) Minoritetsperspektiver i sosialt arbeid [Minority perspectives in Social Work], Universitetsforl, Oslo

Attanapola CT (2013) Migration and health: A literature review of the health of immigrant populations in Norway. Report no 13. NTNU Social Research, Trondheim

Avis M, Elkan R, Patel S et al (2008) Ethnicity and participation in cancer self-help groups. Psycho-Oncol 17:940–947

Balaam MC, Akerjordet K, Lyberg A et al (2013) A qualitative review of migrant women's perceptions of their needs and experiences related to pregnancy and childbirth. J Adv Nurs 69:1919–1930

Blom S (2011) Holdninger til innvandrere og innvandring [Attitudes to immigrant and immigration]. Report, Statistisk sentralbyrå [Statistics Norway], Oslo

Bradby H, Humphris R, Newall D et al (2015) Public health aspects of migrant health: a review of the evidence on health status for refugees and asylum seekers in the European Region. WHO Regional Office for Europe, Copenhagen

Braun V, Clarke V (2006) Using thematic analysis in psychology. Qual Res Psychol 3:77–101

Cargo M, Mercer SL (2008) The value and challenges of participatory research: strengthening its practice. Annu Rev Public Health 29:325–350

Debesay J, Harsløf I, Rechel B et al (2014) Facing diversity under institutional constraints: challenging situations for community nurses when providing care to ethnic minority patients. J Adv Nurs 70:2107–2116

Diaz E, Kumar BN (2018) Health care curricula in multicultural societies. Int J Med Educ 9:42–44

Forland F (2009) Migrasjon og helse: utfordringer og utviklingstrekk [Migration and Health: challenges and trends], Report, Helsedirektoratet [The Norwegian Directorate of Health], Oslo

Giddens A (1984) The constitution of society: outline of the theory of structuration. Polity Press, Cambridge

Goldblatt P, Castedo A, Allen J et al (2023). Rapid review of inequalities in health and wellbeing in Norway since 2014. Report, Institute of Health Equity, University College London, preprint at https://www.instituteofhealthequity.org/resources-reports/rapid-review-of-inequalities-in-health-and-wellbeing-in-norway-since-2014/read-the-full-report.pdf

Hacker K (2017) Community-based participatory research. Sage, London

Hedlund M, Moe A (2010) Redefining relations among minority users and social workers. Eur J Soc Work 13:183–198

Hussaini L, Ezzati RT (2022) Migrasjon og helse i usikre tider [Migration and health in uncertain times]. Tidsskrift for den Norske Lægeforening [The Journal of the Norwegian Medical Association], doi: https://doi.org/10.4045/tidsskr.22.0717

Indseth T, Fretheim A, Ezzati RT et al (2021) Koronapandemien og innvandrerbefolkningene, vurderinger og erfaringer. [The Corona pandemic and immigrant populations, assessments and experiences]. Report, Folkehelseinstituttet [Norwegian Institute of Public Health], Oslo

Isaacs SA, Roman N, Carlson S (2020) Fostering family resilience: a community participatory action research perspective. Child Care Pract 26:358–372

Jenum AK, Holme I, Graff-Iversen S et al (2005) Ethnicity and sex are strong determinants of diabetes in an urban Western society: implications for prevention. Diabetologia 48:435–439

Kale E, Hjelde K, Gele A (2018) 6.10-P3A scoping review study on mental health challenges of immigrants to Norway. Eur J Pub Health 28. https://doi.org/10.1093/eurpub/cky048.210

Kasper J, Stensdal L-A, Kienlin S et al (2022) New status report from Norway: implementation of patient involvement in Norwegian health care. Z Evid Fortbild Qual Gesundhwes 171:105–112

Kinnunen TI, Richardsen KR, Sletner L et al (2019) Ethnic differences in body mass index trajectories from 18 years to postpartum in a population-based cohort of pregnant women in Norway. BMJ Open 9:e022640–e022640. https://doi.org/10.1136/bmjopen-2018-022640

Kumar BN, Holmboe-Ottesen G, Lien N et al (2004) Ethnic differences in body mass index and associated factors of adolescents from minorities in Oslo, Norway: a cross-sectional study. Public Health Nutr 7:999–1008

Le C, Finbråten HS, Pettersen KS et al (2021) Helsekompetansen i fem utvalgte innvandrerpopulasjoner i Norge: Pakistan, Polen, Somalia, Tyrkia og Vietnam. Befolkningens helsekompetanse II. [Health literacy in five selected immigrant populations in Norway: Pakistan, Poland, Somalia, Turkey and Vietnam. The population's health literacy no.II], Helsedirektoratet [The Norwegian Directorate of Health], Oslo

Lebano A, Hamed S, Bradby H et al (2020) Migrants' and refugees' health status and healthcare in Europe: a scoping literature review. BMC Public Health 20:1039–1039

Mehrara L, Gjernes TKO, Young S (2022) Immigrant women's experiences with Norwegian maternal health services: implications for policy and practice. Int J Qual Stud Health Well-Being 17:–2066256

Moe A, Hedlund M (2019) Rethinking research in south Sámi communities. In: Henriksen JE, Ida Hydle I, Kramvig B (eds) Recognition, reconciliation and restoration: applying a decolonized understanding in social work and healing processes. Orkana Akademisk, Stamsund

Norwegian Health Directorate (2021) Helsekompetanse [Health literacy]. Available via Norwegian Directorate of Health. https://www.helsedirektoratet.no/tema/helsekompetanse. Accessed 7 May 2023

Nutbeam D (2000) Health literacy as a public health goal: a challenge for contemporary health education and communication strategies into the 21st century. Health Promot Int 15(3):259–267

Solbjør M, Steinsbekk A (2011) Patient participation in hospital wards—health personnel's experience. Tidsskrift for den Norske laegeforening: tidsskrift for praktisk medicin, ny raekke 131:130–131

Spilker, RS, Aambø, A, Indseth T (2009) Tilstandsrapport: minoritetshelsefeltet i Norge [Minority health field condition report in Norway]. Healthnet, state of the art report (SOAR)], NAKMI report, Oslo

Stalheim AM, Iversen MM, Jenum AK et al (2023) Seasonal variation in gestational diabetes mellitus among women in Norway: a national population-based study. BMJ Open 13:e063725–e063725. https://doi.org/10.1136/bmjopen-2022-063725

Statistic Norway [SSB] (2023) Immigrants and Norwegian-born to immigrant parents. https://www.ssb.no/en/befolkning/innvandrere/statistikk/innvandrere-og-norskfodte-med-innvandrerforeldre. Accessed 15 Oct 2023

Thurston WE, Vissandjée B (2005) An ecological model for understanding culture as a determinant of women's health. Crit Public Health 15:229–242

Varvin S, Aasland OG (2009) Legers forhold til flyktningpasienten [Doctors' relationship with the refugee patient]. Tidsskr Nor Laegeforen [The Journal of the Norwegian Medical Association] 129:1488–1490

Viken B, Lyberg A, Severinsson E (2015) Maternal health coping strategies of migrant women in Norway. Nurs Res Pract 2015:878040–878011

Zhao Y (2017) Health party from concept to practice: follow-up research report on the women's network NOOR's pilot project 'women's health in Nordland—empowerment through health promotion education [Helseparty fra konsept til praksis. Rapport av følgeforskning på kvinnenettverket Noors pilotprosjekt "Kvinnehelse i Nordland—empowerment gjennom helsefremmende allmenndannelse"]. R&D report no.17, Nord University, Bodø

Zhao Y, Gjernes T, Hedlund M (2021) Exploring participation and interaction in a bottom-up health promotion program for migrant women in Norway. Qual Health Res 31:691–702

Chapter 11
The Role of Health Literacy and Care Pathways in the Provision of Palliative Care and Patient-Centred Care: A Discussion Paper

Amaia Urrizola, Tonje Lundeby, Marianne Hjermstad, Luc Deliens, Augusto Caraceni, Marie Fallon, and Stein Kaasa

Abstract Palliative care is more than end-of-life care. It addresses the well-being of patients living with a disease across physical, psychological, social, and existential dimensions. Aligned with the principles of palliative care, patient-centred care is defined as "providing care that is respectful of, and responsive to, individual patient preferences, needs and values". As such, both palliative and patient-centred care are undoubtedly aligned with the Sustainable Development Goals of good health and well-being, and reduced inequalities. Despite recommendations from the WHO and others for its integration throughout the healthcare continuum, palliative care is still commonly perceived as end-of-life care only and is not routinely integrated. This misconception along with social, economic, commercial, and organisational barriers impede its seamless integration in health care. Health literacy is crucial to correct misconceptions and empower patients and caregivers to advocate for appropriate care contributing to good health and reduced inequalities.

In this chapter, we explore how health literacy can be improved, how individual tailoring of the clinical communication according to the patient's health literacy can ensure that the patient voice is heard, and the role of standardised care pathways as a proposed strategy to ensure quality cancer care with integrated palliative care.

A. Urrizola (✉) · T. Lundeby · M. Hjermstad · S. Kaasa
European Palliative Care Research Centre (PRC), Department of Oncology, Oslo University Hospital, and Institute of Clinical Medicine, University of Oslo, Oslo, Norway

L. Deliens
End-of-Life Care Research Group, Vrije Universiteit Brussel and Ghent University, Brussels, Belgium

A. Caraceni
Università degli studi di Milano, Fondazione IRCCS Istituto Nazionale dei Tumori, Milan, Italy

M. Fallon
Institute of Genetics and Molecular Medicine, University of Edinburgh, Edinburgh, UK

T. Hole et al. (eds.), *Towards Sustainable Good Health and Well-being*,
https://doi.org/10.1007/978-3-031-61810-9_11

Finally, we will present the MyPath project as a potential solution to improved care in patients with cancer. By developing digital patient-centred care pathways and supporting the communication and clinical interactions between the healthcare providers, the patient, and caregivers, MyPath will take into account the patient's health literacy and contribute to the Sustainable Development Goals.

Keywords Cancer care · Palliative care · Patient-centred care · Health literacy · Standardised care pathways · Patient-centred care pathways · MyPath · Implementation

11.1 Relationship Between Palliative Care and Sustainable Development Goals

11.1.1 Definition of Palliative Care

Palliative care has its roots in care provided in hospices (Saunders 2001). When it was first introduced, it was focused on and linked to end-of-life care for patients with cancer. The overall aim was to alleviate the existential and spiritual suffering of patients nearing death, as well as the treatment of symptoms. Over time, this approach has transformed from solely end-of-life care to a broader framework where palliative care is integrated in routine health care and seeks to improve care for patients throughout the disease trajectory. In contrast to traditional provisions of palliative care, this new conception envisions the provision of care alongside life-prolonging and curative treatments (Sepúlveda et al. 2002), also including diagnoses of life-limiting illnesses other than cancer (Fig. 11.1).

This approach is in accordance with the most updated definition of palliative care, which states that:

> Palliative care is the active holistic care of individuals across all ages with serious health-related suffering due to severe illness, and especially of those near the end of life. It aims to improve the quality of life of patients, their families, and their caregivers. (Palliative Care Definition n.d.)

Despite ongoing discussions regarding the content of palliative care, the model of delivery, and terminology (i.e. whether to use the term "palliative care" or "supportive care"), the common goal is always "to improve the patient's quality of life congruent with the patient's preferences" (Ryan et al. 2020). Based on the principles of palliative care (Fig. 11.2), patient-centred care is defined by the Institute of Medicine as "providing care that is respectful of, and responsive to, individual patient preferences, needs and values, and ensuring that patient values guide all clinical decisions" (Schuster et al. 2001). In patient-centred care, the focus is the patient living with the disease, and it recognises the multidimensional aspects of care, which encompass not only medical and physical aspects but also psychological, social, and spiritual factors.

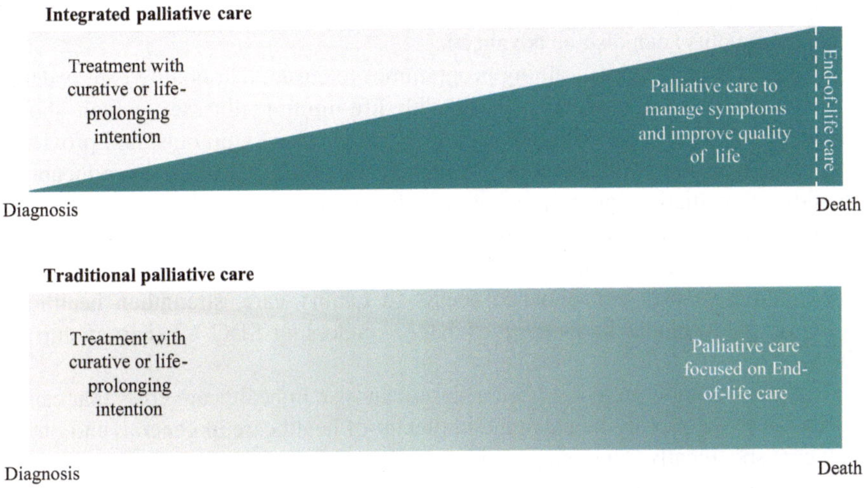

Fig. 11.1 Traditional versus integrated palliative care. Modified from "Integration of oncology and palliative care: a Lancet Oncology Commission" (https://doi.org/10.1016/S1470-2045(18)30415-7)

Principles of Palliative Care

- Focus on quality of life and patient preferences
- Systematic assessment of patient reported outcome measures
- Coordination and continuity of care
- Shared decision-making and advanced care planning
- Appropriate specialist palliative care and hospice referral
- End-of-life care

Fig. 11.2 Principles within a palliative care approach. When palliative is integrated with cancer care, these principles guide the care provided for cancer patients regardless of disease stage. (Author's own figure)

11.1.2 Relationship with the Sustainable Development Goals

Both palliative care and patient-centred care are aligned with the Sustainable Development Goals (SDGs) (Sustainable Development Goals 2023), in particular, the objectives of SDG 3: Good health and well-being and SDG 10: Reduced inequalities. The first emphasises improving the quality of life, alleviating suffering, and supporting patients and their families. The bearing principle of SDG 10 is equity, which is critical in the provision of palliative care (Fact sheet on Palliative Care (WHO) n.d.), and it advocates for reducing disparities in access to health care and improving health outcomes for all patients, regardless of socio-economic status, ethnicity, or religion. Moreover, by providing equitable palliative care that recognises and considers gender-specific needs and cultural sensitivities, SDG 5 (Gender equality) can also be advanced.

Palliative care requires training programmes to ensure that quality care is delivered to all patients, especially those with life-limiting illnesses, which should include communication skills, managing pain and other symptoms, and providing compassionate end-of-life care, thus being aligned with SDG 4 (Quality education). In addition, palliative care requires a multidisciplinary approach and collaboration among healthcare providers, families, and communities. By fostering partnerships between healthcare institutions, governments, NGOs, and community organisations, palliative care can enhance access to quality care, strengthen healthcare systems, and promote knowledge exchange, endorsing SDG 17 (Partnership for the goals).

In the past years, there has been a significant rise in healthcare costs that can be attributed to the rapidly increasing complexity of healthcare in general, and oncology care specifically. The rising costs threatens the sustainability of current healthcare services, especially in the field of cancer care (Schnipper et al. 2012). Patient-centred care that improves symptoms, satisfaction, and other patient-centred outcomes may reduce costs (Kaasa et al. 2017), given less aggressive treatments, and shorter lengths-of-stay in hospital, fewer emergency admissions (May et al. 2018), and better use of resources coherent with the patients' values (Harris and Murray 2013), contributing to SDG 12 (Responsible consumption and production).

11.1.3 Barriers and Lack of Implementation: Problems Faced by Palliative Care

Multiple randomised controlled trials and studies have been conducted and show that early provision of palliative care results in better quality of care, better patient involvement and improves the quality of life, symptoms, and survival while reducing costs at the same time (Kaasa et al. 2018; May et al. 2018; Bajwah et al. 2020). Although the magnitude of the studies was small, a recent Cochrane review concluded that integrated care may still be beneficial to patients and carers (Bajwah et al. 2020). Based on this evidence, international organisations such as the World Health Organization (WHO), the European Society for Medical Oncology (ESMO), and the American Society of Clinical Oncology (ASCO) recommend early integration of palliative care (Kaasa et al. 2018). These recommendations are aligned with the promotion of SDG 3 on Good health and well-being.

In 2018, ESMO proposed a series of key strategies to be undertaken by different stakeholders in order to address SDG 3 for cancer patients. Most of the strategies are focused on tumour-centred care, but the document reinforces the importance of palliative care as well, particularly on strategies for improving access for all patients (Prager et al. 2018).

Despite its evident benefits and endorsed recommendations, palliative care is still commonly associated with end-of-life care and is not routinely integrated in health care. From the point of view of the provision of care, the barriers that impede the integration of palliative care can be grouped into those related to the attitudes towards it, which can be traced back to misconceptions and misunderstandings of what palliative care entails, as well as social, economic, commercial, and organisational barriers for the provision of palliative care (Kaasa et al. 2018; Kaasa et al. 2022). Commercial interests and the dominating focus in society on continuing anti-cancer treatment and curation lead to futile treatments and increased consumption of pharmacological products, thereby challenging responsible consumption (SDG 12). Moreover, this attitude is reinforced by the medical and technological development that in turn increases the demand for treatment, as pointed out later in the chapter, and by the political agenda that promotes and prioritises cancer curation.

In addition, existing inequalities regarding the socio-economic status have an impact in the awareness, access, and use of the different health services, including palliative care. By improving education, and thus health literacy (SDG 4), it will be possible to increase equal access to good health care (SDGs 3, 4, and 10).

In order to overcome these barriers and work towards the integration and promotion of palliative care and patient-centred care, joint collaboration and drive between different stakeholders will be needed (SDG 17).

11.1.3.1 Lack of Awareness and Misconceptions

Patients, Caregivers, and the General Population

In a national survey performed in the United States, up to 70% of the participants indicated that they had never heard of palliative care (Trivedi et al. 2019). Even if the self-reported rates of palliative care knowledge seemed to rise over the years, it did not translate into an accurate understanding of what palliative care is. A study assessing what patient's understood as palliative care indicated that half of the respondents associated palliative care with hospice and end-of-life care (Zhu and Engui 2019).

Currently, most people who have not experienced first- or second-hand what palliative care is or who have not cared for someone with a serious illness struggle to understand the meaning of palliative care (Zimmermann et al. 2016). This is particularly true for patients with low health literacy (for example, those with cultural backgrounds or who speak languages which are different to that of their country of residence or have a lower level of education and lack of experience). Thus, there is a need for more widespread understanding of basic palliative care principles among patients, particularly those who may be less familiar with it due to lower levels of education.

Health Care Providers

However, patients and caregivers are not the only ones who struggle with the concept of palliative care. Healthcare providers frequently consider palliative care as equivalent to end-of-life care, viewing it as "passive and not offering hope" (Kaasa et al. 2022). As a result, healthcare providers working with care and life prolongation are reluctant to make referrals for palliative care.

A systematic review assessing the views of oncologists and haematologists on palliative care referrals showed that making the referral elicited negative emotions in the healthcare providers. Moreover, it identified role conflict, abandonment, rupture of therapeutic alliance, and loss of hope as some of the perceptions that could hinder such referrals (Salins et al. 2020). In other situations, healthcare providers believed that specialist palliative care can be easily provided by any physician or oncologist, and/or they have the self-efficacy to manage palliative care needs (Salins et al. 2020), thus considering a referral unnecessary (Salins et al. 2020; Kaasa et al. 2022).

These attitudes from healthcare providers reflect a lack of organisational health literacy, thus making it more difficult to truly enact shared decision-making and help patients make informed choices.

11.1.3.2 Palliative Care Competes with Tumour-Centred Care

The commercial determinants of health include social, commercial, and economic interests that shape the provision of care (Fig. 11.3).

Society Does Not Want to Talk About Death

We currently live in a society that perceives death as negative and a topic to be avoided, so much so that in the past decades, there has been an argument in the ongoing discussion that Western societies are death-denying societies (Zimmermann 2004). Currently, we consider medicine *"the 'fight' against disease" and death "as having 'lost the battle'"* (Gellie et al. 2015), which, combined with an incessant marketing on staying young and healthy forever, makes talking about dying uncomfortable and also a taboo.

Medicine Taught in Curative Terms: Conquer Disease and Defeat Death

Medicine is frequently taught and framed in curative terms. The main goal is to cure the patient and conquer the disease, hence perceiving the inability to cure a failure, which in turn can lead to therapeutic obstinacy and futile treatments. In oncology, the erroneous perception of regarding ineffective treatment as a failure is predominant, thereby impeding the discontinuation of futile treatment, even when it

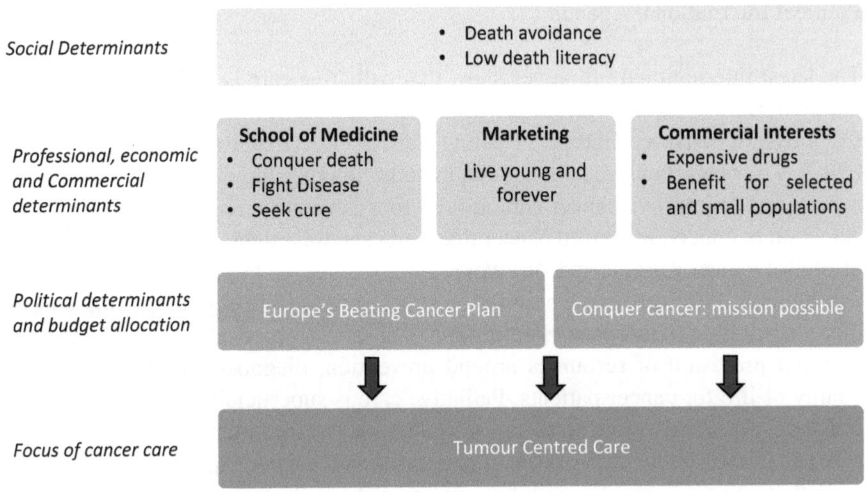

Fig. 11.3 Commercial determinants of health. The interaction between social, commercial, economic, and political interests that lead to an increased focus on tumour-centred care. (Author's own figure)

provides no expected benefits and high toxicity. Provision of anti-cancer treatment and intensive end-of-life care is not in line with recommendations for good clinical practice by ASCO, WHO, and ESMO, and it leads to spiralling societal and health care costs and negative patient outcomes, as well as increasing demands for a cure from society at large.

Medical students are taught to cure the disease and less to care for the patient; especially, students receive very little, if any, training regarding end-of-life care. Moreover, when palliative care is understood as end-of-life care or a referral that takes place when "nothing else can be done", clinicians consider the referral a therapeutic failure (Salins et al. 2020) and do not consider palliative care because it may entail "admitting defeat".

Commercial Interests

Commercial interests also lead to an increased focus on the development and promotion of new and expensive drugs that benefit highly selected groups of patients. The tendency to oversee or underestimate the side effects of anti-cancer treatment, paired with marketing initiatives that claim that most cancers can be cured, reinforces the initiation of futile treatments (Kaasa et al. 2022), which does not adhere to a responsible consumption (SDG 12). New therapies have improved the survival rates of many cancers. These improvements have strengthened the perception that cancer can be "cured forever". As a result, a stronger than ever focus on curation, prolongation of life, and medical advances prevails nowadays, resulting in funding being disproportionately allocated to tumour-centred care.

Political International Agenda

The latest international initiatives show that palliative care is still not a priority on the international agenda for improving cancer outcomes. In 2021, the European Commission delivered Europe's Beating Cancer Plan (EBCP) (EU, EC 2021). The EBCP is a comprehensive strategy that includes ten flagship initiatives and supporting actions to improve cancer care around four key action areas: prevention, early detection of cancer, improved cancer diagnosis and treatment, and improved quality of life for cancer patients and survivors.

Likewise, the European Commission's Mission on Cancer (Conquering cancer: mission possible) (European Commission et al. 2020) proposal covers the information and provision of resources around prevention, diagnosis and treatment, and quality of life for cancer patients. Palliative care is superficially mentioned in both initiatives; however, both plans fail to recognise the important role that palliative care has in the quality care of cancer patients (Caraceni and Apolone 2021).

Palliative care competes with tumour-centred care in terms of research but also in care provision. In the clinical environment, healthcare providers are influenced by the commercial determinants of health, and the societal, economical, and political spheres that promote tumour-centred care. As a result, the model that prevails is the tumour-centred care approach that focuses on explaining the disease and treatment options without considering the person living with the disease.

In addition, a tumour-centred approach combined with misconceptions about palliative care perpetuates the traditional palliative care approach (Fig. 11.4). In this setting, referrals to palliative care occur too late since it is considered passive and limited to end-of-life care, offered when there is no hope, with most clinicians

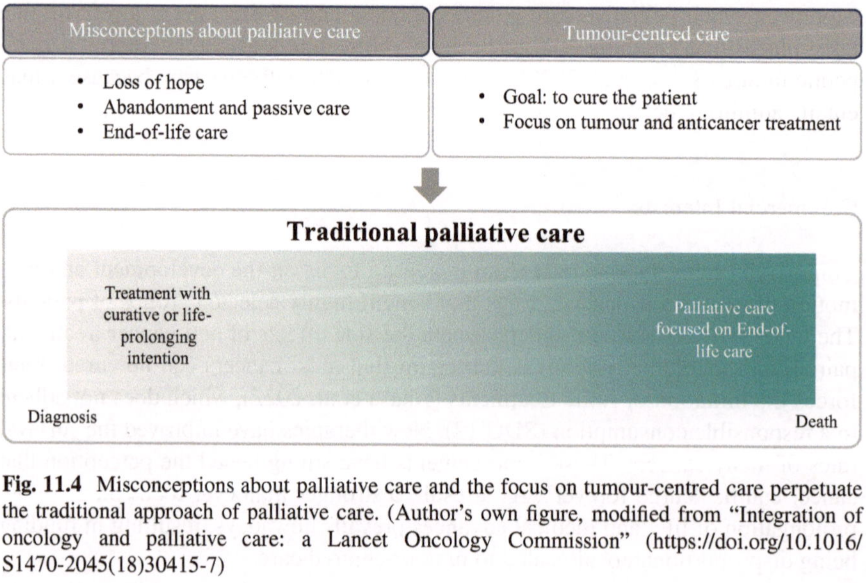

Fig. 11.4 Misconceptions about palliative care and the focus on tumour-centred care perpetuate the traditional approach of palliative care. (Author's own figure, modified from "Integration of oncology and palliative care: a Lancet Oncology Commission" (https://doi.org/10.1016/S1470-2045(18)30415-7)

experiencing feelings of abandoning the patient. Most importantly, they leave a high number of patients who need palliative care "unattended", and with suboptimal consideration to their needs, falling short in terms of providing care for a good health (SDG 3).

To address this gap, public health demands, organisation of care, and priorities need to align with palliative care principles. Implementing palliative care into clinical practice will require a concerted effort (SDG 17) by health care providers, policymakers, and society as a whole to improve health literacy and an understanding of palliative care, prioritise patient-centred care, and advocate for sustainable development.

11.2 Health Literacy: Why It Is Important for Palliative Care

Low levels of health literacy have been identified among patients, caregivers, and healthcare professionals and have been linked to poor health outcomes, particularly in relation to palliative care, perpetuating health inequalities (Christensen 2016). An improved education (SDG 4) and health literacy, particularly related to palliative care, health, treatment, prognosis, and death, can contribute to reducing inequalities (SDG 10) and the better use of the healthcare services and palliative care in some specific elements. It can facilitate necessary discussions about death in our society and increase the understanding of what palliative care is and its role beyond end-of-life care. Health literacy can also improve the communication and shared decision-making between the healthcare providers and the patients, thus empowering patients to demand the right care for good health (SDG 3) and focus on what matters most when life "does not last forever" by engaging in advance care planning, which in turn supports a responsible consumption (SDG 12).

11.2.1 Talking About Death

Talking about poor prognosis, death, and dying, including preferences, hopes, and fears, is viewed as one of the most challenging discussions by healthcare providers in palliative care. Uncertainty about a given prognosis, lack of training, fear of negatively impacting the patient, and patient "readiness" to discuss these topics seem to be the most common barriers. Further, it represents a difficult personal situation for the individual care provider. However, in this context, more emphasis should be put on the positive impacts on the quality and satisfaction with care experienced by patients after they have end-of-life care discussions with the healthcare providers (Brighton and Bristowe 2016).

Developing education and literacy about death in the community through education activities and learning experiences can help normalise end-of-life (Noonan et al. 2016). Death literacy can be defined as:

> The knowledge and skills that people need to make it possible to gain access to, understand, and make informed choices about end-of-life and death care options. People and communities with high levels of death literacy have context specific knowledge about the death system and the ability to put that knowledge into practice. (Patterson and Hazelwood 2022)

It has been suggested that providing informal care at home at the end-of-life can deepen the understanding and contributes to changes in attitudes and social actions around death and dying (Noonan et al. 2016). Caring and being involved in end-of-life care is a learning experience. It has been considered by the carers and their networks as a catalyst for learning about end-of-life care (Leonard et al. 2020). Moreover, community approaches in palliative care (considering the community as equal partners in the long and complex task of providing quality health care at the end of life) can improve the death literacy of our population and hence empower people to have more active and supportive roles in palliative care (Johansson and Eriksson 2023).

Finally, an open public discussion about what is meant by the ordinary concept of death can help both patients and clinicians to talk "openly" and encourage patients and families to participate in discussions about treatment goals (Gellie et al. 2015; Noonan et al. 2016).

11.2.2 Understanding Palliative Care: Perceptions

Being aware of all that can be achieved by palliative care throughout the trajectory of the disease can help both patients and healthcare providers understand why early referrals to palliative care are beneficial. It is important to bear in mind that the referral should not imply a separate care. Instead, it should translate into a closer collaboration with oncologists, other healthcare providers, and community care, with the patient at the centre.

From a patient's perspective, low levels of knowledge of palliative care can lead to misunderstandings and confusion. When patients have not experienced or been informed sufficiently about the benefits of patient-centred care and palliative care (or caring for someone with a serious illness), they tend to associate palliative care with end-of-life care and react with fear and hopelessness upon the referral or involvement of palliative care during treatment. On the contrary, patients who have a reasonable understanding and/or have experienced what palliative care can do, have a more positive attitude (Zimmermann et al. 2016). Likewise, if healthcare providers understand and accept that palliative care is complementary and beneficial, also to the actual outcomes of tumour-centred care, they may be less reluctant to refer to specialist care when needed, integrating palliative care in the routine care of cancer patients (Fig. 11.5).

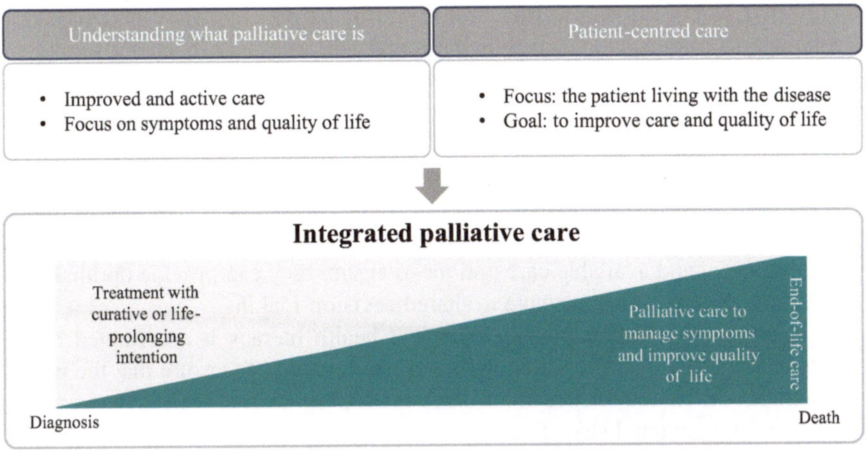

Fig. 11.5 Accurate perceptions of palliative care and a patient-centred approach facilitate the integration of palliative care. (Author's own figure, Modified from "Integration of oncology and palliative care: a Lancet Oncology Commission" (https://doi.org/10.1016/S1470-2045(18)30415-7)

11.2.3 Communication and Shared Decision-Making

Effective communication and shared decision-making are essential for the delivery of high-quality palliative care.

Limited health literacy can impact the provision of care due to misconceptions about cancer as well as ineffective communication with the healthcare providers involved (Koay et al. 2012). In addition, these patients may struggle with filling in questionnaires or reporting outcomes, as well as reading, understanding, and applying information about their health and health care. Challenges in understanding their prognosis and treatment recommendations can impact their ability to make informed decisions. As a result, patients with limited health literacy may make "inappropriate" demands, receive unnecessary interventions, and adhere poorly to their recommended treatment.

Low levels of health literacy are associated with poor health outcomes. Patients who have low health literacy tend to have higher rates of hospitalisation and visits to the emergency room and fail to take medications appropriately. This includes not only poor adherence to treatment but also misuse of the medication, alongside worse symptom control, which is especially relevant regarding opioid use and pain control (Rogers et al. 2020).

Not only does limited health literacy lead to poor health outcomes but in addition it can perpetuate health inequalities (Christensen 2016). Patient empowerment, which involves an active role for patients in terms of their health, requires health literacy so that they can demand or request appropriate care and truly enact shared decision-making.

Informal caregivers play a crucial role in caring for patients. They tend to be family members or others who engage in the actual care work and social and emotional support and share the disease experience with patients (Gardiner et al. 2020). However, a study assessing the health literacy of caregivers found that many reported that they encountered difficulties in managing areas related to the use of medication and symptom recognition (Metin et al. 2019).

Due to their active and pivotal role of informal caregivers, it is of utmost importance that they have a clear understanding of the palliative care principles, the disease prognosis, and available care options to ensure they can provide optimal care, support the patient, and contribute to shared decision-making.

It is paramount that the patient's level of health literacy is ascertained by the healthcare providers at the beginning of the care process, to ensure that the patient understands the characteristics of the disease, the prognosis, as well as the treatment objectives and potential side effects.

11.2.4 Advance Care Planning

Advance care planning provides patients with the means of ensuring that their preferences and wishes are identified and recorded, thus guiding any treatment and care when life is limited, and the disease is incurable. Advance care planning positively impacts the quality of end-of-life care and leads to a decrease in futile treatments and life-sustaining treatments: it prevents hospitalisations and increases the use of palliative care (Brinkman-Stoppelenburg et al. 2014). Additionally, it is viewed as a way of continuing shared decision-making even when the patient is no longer able to do so. The fulfilment of advanced care planning usually takes place after an event (diagnosis, recurrence, hospital or hospice admission, etc.) that marks a transition in the status of the patient's health (Lund et al. 2015). However, it is still not routinely included in daily care. Time constraints are one of the most commonly claimed reasons by healthcare providers, coupled with insecurity, lack of education, and absence of training in this regard (Blackwood et al. 2019). Although there is limited data, advance care planning interventions tailored for limited health literacy patients increase knowledge regarding advance directives, preference for comfort care, and completion of advanced care planning documentation (Houlihan et al. 2022).

In conclusion, education (SDG 4) and health literacy play a crucial role in improving palliative care and patient-centred care provision. A collaborative effort (SDG 17) should be made to improve health literacy among patients, caregivers, and healthcare professionals to ensure effective communication and shared decision-making, and therefore improve health outcomes and contribute to well-being (SDG 3).

11.3 Improving Health Literacy

Improving health literacy can help reduce healthcare inequalities (SDG 10), as users with good health literacy can better navigate the healthcare system and access appropriate services and care regardless of socio-economic status. One step towards improving health literacy is the need for accessible and understandable patient education (SDG 4) resources in palliative care and oncology. Although the Internet is a popular source of health information, and frequently used by patients and carers, if misused or misinterpreted, it can be misleading. Moreover, when assessed, over 85% of available patient education materials about palliative care are above the recommended degree of difficulty for ensuring understanding (Prabhu et al. 2017). Patient education materials need to be designed at an appropriate level of complexity, as many patients may struggle to understand complex medical terminology and concepts.

This section provides an overview of some strategies that healthcare providers can use to help patients with limited health literacy access the best care (SDG 3), such as recognising the patient's health literacy, using plain language and metaphors, and assessing understanding.

In order to facilitate the implementation of these strategies, organisational changes and collaboration between different stakeholders (SDG 17) will be necessary to ensure the appropriate training of healthcare providers at the undergraduate and postgraduate levels. These changes and collaboration can contribute to (increasing) organisational health literacy which in turn will facilitate the enhancement of patients' health literacy and support patients with lower levels of health literacy.

11.3.1 Patients' Health Literacy: Recognising and Adapting

To optimize the delivery of appropriate care, it is crucial to recognize when patients and their caregivers have limited health literacy. Healthcare providers tend to overestimate patients' health literacy, missing chances to help patients understand medical information (Kelly and Haidet 2007; Christensen 2016). Implementing routine health literacy screening and assessment tools in clinical practice can help clinicians adapt communication strategies accordingly. A few simple questions about the patient's level of knowledge about the disease may be effective and can set the agenda for further information. Moreover, it does not take much time and may prove effective during the actual consultation and follow-up.

11.3.1.1 Plain Language and Visual Aids

Difficulty in understanding medical terminology is one of the most frequent indicators of limited health literacy. Utilising plain language can help patients and caregivers better understand complex health information and engage in shared decision-making (Rudd et al. 2004). Thus, when meeting with patients with lower levels of health literacy, the use of plain language (using simple words, short sentences, and clear explanations) and avoiding technical and medical jargon should be prioritised.

Providing materials that are appropriate and tailored to a patient's specific needs can further enhance understanding. It is important that healthcare providers invest time with the patient and caregivers, ensuring their understanding after they have read the information. Special attention should be given to providing effective communication with patients from different cultural backgrounds which requires an understanding of the patient's cultural beliefs, values, and practices. Culturally sensitive communication involves showing respect, avoiding assumptions, and being open to learning from the patient about their unique perspective (Betancourt 2006).

Metaphors and visual aids (such as diagrams, charts, and illustrations) can help patients with limited health literacy better understand complex health information. Metaphors can prove useful particularly for supporting and promoting the understanding of challenging discussions. Zimmerman et al. designed the illustrated metaphor "palliative care is the umbrella, not the rain" as a tool for oncologists to better explain to patients what palliative care is, and as such, facilitate referrals. Their work, published in *JAMA Oncology*, aims to address frequent misconceptions that patients (and healthcare providers) have against palliative care, and that frequently act as a barrier to early referrals (Zimmermann and Mathews 2022).

A useful method for assessing the patient's understanding of the information would be asking patients to repeat back to the clinician, in their own words, the information or instructions given to them. This method known as teach-back method allows clinicians to make any necessary clarifications, and it has shown to improve treatment adherence, self-efficacy, and disease-specific knowledge (Ha Dinh et al. 2016).

11.3.2 Assessing Understanding: Encouraging Patients and Families to Ask Questions and Seek Clarification

Patient and caregivers with limited health literacy are, frequently, reluctant to ask questions (Parikh et al. 1996; Katz et al. 2007). Healthcare providers should actively encourage patients and families to ask questions and seek clarification about their care and treatment options. They can prompt patients by asking open-ended questions or providing examples of relevant enquiries. This approach not only helps patients and families better understand their care but also allows healthcare professionals to identify areas of confusion and tailor their communication(s) accordingly.

Improved communication between interdisciplinary teams, including medical professionals, social workers, and patient navigators, can help support patients with limited health literacy. These teams can work together to address the diverse needs of patients and their families, ensuring that they receive comprehensive care and are empowered to make informed decisions about their treatment options.

11.3.3 Improving Communication and Shared Decision-Making: Training and Education Healthcare Providers

"The art of communication is to use the right tool for the right person at the right time" (Hui et al. 2018). Once limited health literacy is recognised, there are evidence-based approaches that healthcare providers can use to promote communication and shared decision-making. Healthcare providers identify communication difficulties, lack of training, and limited resources as major obstacles to providing effective palliative care (Kaasa et al. 2018).

Disclosing the disease is incurable, discussing prognosis, and palliative care referrals are conversations that physicians struggle to have and are associated with negative emotions and experiences (Brighton and Bristowe 2016). However, it can become easier for healthcare providers to tackle these needed conversations with patients when they have the right communication tools and guidance. Hence, clinicians should receive specific training regarding known effective techniques for improving communication (i.e. COMFORT communication training (Wittenberg et al. 2018)). This training should cover theoretical and practical aspects and should also be part of the curricula in all healthcare education programmes. Blended training programmes for clinicians have been shown to improve communication with patients with limited health literacy and increase patients' understanding of their situation and involvement in decision-making (Noordman et al. 2022).

11.4 Can Digital Patient-Centred Care Pathways Lower the Bar for Patients and Caregivers with Limited Health Literacy?

There is a need for a new clinical approach with patient-centred care as the cornerstone, resulting in more patient involvement and an individual approach tailored to the patient's needs. In patient-centred care, the focus is patients living with cancer as well as the disease, incorporating patient-centred and tumour-centred approaches.

Patient-centred care does not only benefit patients but also benefits families, caregivers, the community, and healthcare systems.

Standardised clinical pathways have been proposed as a solution to implement patient-centred care in routine cancer care and are recommended by EU policy to ensure quality care (Albreht et al. 2017) through the continuum of cancer care; from screening and diagnosis, through treatment, to long-term monitoring and support in survivors and end-of-life care. Clinical pathways (European Pathway Association n.d.) represent a "set" of detailed steps that guide complex, and often multidisciplinary, decision-making processes, including provision and organisation of care processes within a care plan for a well-defined group of patients during a specific period. As such, these pathways provide a treatment plan for a given patient population and support the integration of clinical guidelines into local protocols and clinical practice. The pathway can be adjusted according to time or criteria-based progression.

Implementing pathways that combine the systematic assessment of patient-reported outcome measures (PROMs) with appropriate evidence-based care plans can result in improved patient-centred care. The use of PROMs in routine clinical care, with special attention to ensure understanding by patients with limited health literacy, is recommended by ESMO for all patients during systemic cancer treatment (Di Maio et al. 2022). PROMs aim to assess symptoms, functions, and health-related quality of life of the patients (Basch et al. 2017). Systematic retrieval of PROMs brings the patient's voice directly into the consultation and provides a clearer picture of the patient's needs and burdens. It is a multidimensional strategy that also takes health literacy into account because it listens to the patient, adapts to the patient's needs, and includes actions to be discussed and agreed upon.

Funded by the EU's Horizon Europe programme, MyPath (Cordis Europa 2022) is an implementation study that intends to incorporate patient-centred care into routine cancer care. To achieve it, the project aims to develop a digital solution based on patient-centred care pathways that combines a systematic PROMs retrieval ("listening to the patient's voice") paired with evidence-based recommendations. The implementation of pathways using digital solutions provides room for individualised care, adapting to the patient's needs and preferences.

In MyPath, the established patient-centred pathways will support and standardise the optimal clinical process in daily practice. By pairing the digital PROMs assessment with the best available evidence for management, MyPath will ensure that the recommendations are tailored to each individual patient. Furthermore, the solution will aim to improve patient participation by providing the necessary tools for appropriate shared decision-making based on the patient's needs, values, and preferences.

The implementation science methodology is the cornerstone of the project and will warrant that the patient-centred pathways are followed and incorporated into daily practice. This means that today's clinical work processes must be adapted to a "new era" where modern Health Information Technology sets the framework for implementation.

In order to ensure appropriate communication and patient engagement, the patient's health literacy should be assessed throughout the process. MyPath can assess the health literacy of the patient and provide the appropriate recommendations to guarantee that the healthcare providers are aware of it and adapt their communication skills. Moreover, for patients with limited health literacy, MyPath can also play a role improving their health literacy levels and care by:

- Bringing the patient voice to the clinical consultation. By systematically collecting PROMs adapted to patients with different backgrounds and levels of health literacy, MyPath aims to bring the patient's voice to the consultation, making sure all needs are assessed and addressed.
- Guiding healthcare providers to provide patient-centred care and engage in shared decision-making. Combined with information from the clinical consultation and the electronic health records, the solution suggests patient-centred care pathways that the clinicians will share with the patient, ensuring shared decision-making.
- Guiding patients and caregivers by:
- Providing reliable resources and sources of information concerning the disease, prognosis, and treatment options.
- Providing easily understandable recommendations for self-management.

MyPath will contribute to improved care for patients with incurable diseases. These patients experience a high symptom burden and unmet needs even at the time of diagnosis (Vogt et al. 2021). By assessing systematically symptoms, functions, and quality of life, as well as providing decision support for the clinicians, MyPath can help identify and provide patient-centred care for all patients, with referrals to palliative care when needed.

11.5 Conclusion

Palliative care is much more than end-of-life care. Focused on the physical, psychological, social, and existential well-being of the patient living with the disease, palliative care has been shown to improve symptom control, quality of care, and survival of patients when initiated early in the course of the disease. Moreover, it is aligned with several of the Sustainable Development Goals established by the United Nations – especially the ones concerning good health and well-being, and reduced inequalities.

Despite its benefits and the recommendations endorsed by international bodies, palliative care is still not routinely integrated in health care. Health literacy is a pivotal factor in palliative care, since it influences patients' proper understanding of what is palliative care, as well as improved communication and shared decision-making that can lead to the appropriate care provision.

There are different solutions that healthcare providers can incorporate to assess and tailor clinical communications and decision-making for patients with limited literacy that can improve individual health literacy. In addition to these individual efforts, organisational changes and collaborations need to take place to ensure organisational health literacy. Clinical pathways support the integration of clinical guidelines and recommendations into clinical practice and have been proposed as a solution to ensure access to good care and quality care for patients.

MyPath, as an implementation project aiming to develop innovative digital patient-centred care pathways, will take health literacy into account to guide and tailor the communication and clinical interactions between the healthcare providers, the patient, and the caregivers and provide patients and healthcare providers with appropriate resources to improve shared decision-making, self-management, and treatment adherence. As a result, MyPath can contribute to both patient and organisational health literacy.

References

Albreht T, Kiasuwa R, Van den Bulcke M (2017) European guide on quality improvement in comprehensive cancer control

Bajwah S et al (2020) The effectiveness and cost-effectiveness of hospital-based specialist palliative care for adults with advanced illness and their caregivers. Cochrane Datab Syst Rev 2020(9). https://doi.org/10.1002/14651858.CD012780.pub2

Basch E et al (2017) Overall survival results of a trial assessing patient-reported outcomes for symptom monitoring during routine cancer treatment. JAMA J Am Med Assoc 318(2):197–198. https://doi.org/10.1001/jama.2017.7156

Betancourt JR (2006) Cultural competency-providing quality care to diverse populations. Consult Pharm 21(12):988–995

Blackwood DH et al (2019) Barriers to advance care planning with patients as perceived by nurses and other healthcare professionals: a systematic review. J Clin Nurs 28(23–24):4276–4297. https://doi.org/10.1111/jocn.15049

Brighton LJ, Bristowe K (2016) Communication in palliative care: talking about the end of life, before the end of life. Postgrad Med J 92(1090):466–470. https://doi.org/10.1136/postgradmedj-2015-133368

Brinkman-Stoppelenburg A, Rietjens JAC, Van Der Heide A (2014) The effects of advance care planning on end-of-life care: a systematic review. Palliat Med 28(8):1000–1025. https://doi.org/10.1177/0269216314526272

Caraceni A, Apolone G (2021) 'Conquer cancer for everyone', Lancet Oncol, 22(5), pp. 583–584. 10.1016/S1470-2045(21)00059-0

Christensen D (2016) The impact of health literacy on palliative care outcomes. J Hosp Palliat Nurs 18(6):544–549. https://doi.org/10.1097/NJH.0000000000000292

Cordis Europa (2022). Available at https://cordis.europa.eu/project/id/101057514. Accessed 13 Dec 2023

Di Maio M et al (2022) The role of patient-reported outcome measures in the continuum of cancer clinical care: ESMO clinical practice guideline ☆. Ann Oncol 33(9):878–892. https://doi.org/10.1016/j.annonc.2022.04.007

EU, EC (2021) Communication from the Commission to the European Parliament and the Council – Europe's Beating Cancer Plan

European Commission et al (2020) Conquering cancer: mission possible. Publications Office. https://doi.org/10.2777/284352

European Pathway Association (n.d.) Available at: https://e-p-a.org/care-pathways/. Accessed 28 Aug 2023

Fact sheet on Palliative Care (WHO) (n.d.) Available at: https://www.who.int/news-room/fact-sheets/detail/palliative-care. Accessed 29 Mar 2023

Gardiner C et al (2020) Equity and the financial costs of informal caregiving in palliative care: a critical debate. BMC Palliat Care 19(1):1–7. https://doi.org/10.1186/s12904-020-00577-2

Gellie A et al (2015) Death: a foe to be conquered? Questioning the paradigm. Age Ageing 44(1):7–10. https://doi.org/10.1093/AGEING/AFU116

Ha Dinh TT et al (2016) The effectiveness of the teach-back method on adherence and self-management in health education for people with chronic disease: a systematic review. JBI Database System Rev Implement Rep 14(1):210–247. https://doi.org/10.11124/jbisrir-2016-2296

Harris I, Murray SA (2013) Can palliative care reduce futile treatment? A systematic review. BMJ Support Palliat Care 3(4):389–398. https://doi.org/10.1136/bmjspcare-2012-000343

Houlihan MCK et al (2022) A review of clinical trials of advance care planning interventions adapted for limited health literacy. Palliat Support Care 20(4):593–599. https://doi.org/10.1017/S1478951521001152

Hui D, Zhukovsky DS, Bruera E (2018) Serious illness conversations: paving the road with metaphors. Oncologist 23(6):730–733. https://doi.org/10.1634/theoncologist.2017-0448

Johansson T, Eriksson LE (2023) Factors associated with death literacy among Swedish adults: a cross-sectional exploratory study

Kaasa S et al (2017) Integraton between oncology and palliatve care: a plan for the next decade? Tumori 103(1):1–8. https://doi.org/10.5301/tj.5000602

Kaasa S et al (2018) Integration of oncology and palliative care: a lancet oncology commission. Lancet Oncol 19(11):e588–e653. https://doi.org/10.1016/S1470-2045(18)30415-7

Kaasa BS, Hjermstad MJ, Sjøgren P (2022) Commercial and social determinants in. 28(2):22–27

Katz MG et al (2007) Patient literacy and question-asking behavior during the medical encounter: a mixed-methods analysis. J Gen Intern Med 22(6):782–786. https://doi.org/10.1007/s11606-007-0184-6

Kelly PA, Haidet P (2007) Physician overestimation of patient literacy: a potential source of health care disparities. Patient Educ Couns 66(1):119–122. https://doi.org/10.1016/j.pec.2006.10.007

Koay K, Schofield P, Jefford M (2012) Importance of health literacy in oncology. Asia Pac J Clin Oncol 8(1):14–23. https://doi.org/10.1111/j.1743-7563.2012.01522.x

Leonard R et al. (2020) Death literacy index: a report on its development

Lund S, Richardson A, May C (2015) Barriers to advance care planning at the end of life: an explanatory systematic review of implementation studies. PLoS One 10(2):1–15. https://doi.org/10.1371/journal.pone.0116629

May P et al (2018) 'Economics of palliative care for hospitalized adults with serious illness: a meta-analysis', *JAMA*. Intern Med 178(6):820–829. https://doi.org/10.1001/jamainternmed.2018.0750

Metin S, Demirci H, Metin AT (2019) Effect of health literacy of caregivers on survival rates of patients under palliative care. Scand J Caring Sci 33(3):669–676. https://doi.org/10.1111/scs.12662

Noonan K et al (2016) Developing death literacy. Progr Palliat Care 24(1):31–35. https://doi.org/10.1080/09699260.2015.1103498

Noordman J et al (2022) "A basic understanding"; evaluation of a blended training programme for healthcare providers in hospital-based palliative care to improve communication with patients with limited health literacy. BMC Med Educ 22(1):1–11. https://doi.org/10.1186/s12909-022-03685-0

Palliative Care Definition (n.d.) Available at: https://hospicecare.com/what-we-do/projects/consensus-based-definition-of-palliative-care/definition/. Accessed 27 Apr 2023

Parikh NS et al (1996) Shame and health literacy: the unspoken connection. Patient Educ Couns 27(1):33–39. https://doi.org/10.1016/0738-3991(95)00787-3

Patterson RM, Hazelwood MA (2022) Developing end of life literacy through public education. In: Oxford textbook of public health palliative care. Oxford University Press, pp 126–136

Prabhu AV et al (2017) Online palliative care and oncology patient education resources through Google: do they meet national health literacy recommendations? Pract Radiat Oncol 7(5):306–310. https://doi.org/10.1016/j.prro.2017.01.013

Prager GW et al (2018) Global cancer control: responding to the growing burden, rising costs and inequalities in access. ESMO Open 3(2). https://doi.org/10.1136/esmoopen-2017-000285

Rogers AH et al (2020) Health literacy, opioid misuse, and pain experience among adults with chronic pain. Pain Med (United States) 21(4):670–676. https://doi.org/10.1093/PM/PNZ062

Rudd RE et al (2004) Rewriting public health information in plain language. J Health Commun 9(3):195–206. https://doi.org/10.1080/10810730490447039

Ryan S et al (2020) Evolving definitions of palliative care: upstream migration or confusion? Curr Treat Options in Oncol 21(3):20. https://doi.org/10.1007/s11864-020-0716-4

Salins N et al (2020) How views of oncologists and haematologists impacts palliative care referral: a systematic review. BMC Palliat Care 19(1):1–19. https://doi.org/10.1186/s12904-020-00671-5

Saunders C (2001) The evolution of palliative care. J R Soc Med 94:430–432

Schnipper LE et al (2012) American society of clinical oncology identifies five key opportunities to improve care and reduce costs: the top five list for oncology. J Clin Oncol 30(14):1715–1724. https://doi.org/10.1200/JCO.2012.42.8375

Schuster MA et al (2001) The quality of health care in the United States: a review of articles since 1987, crossing the quality chasm: a new health system for the 21st century

Sepúlveda C et al (2002) Palliative care: the world health organization's global perspective. J Pain Symptom Manag 24(2):91–96. https://doi.org/10.1016/S0885-3924(02)00440-2

Sustainable Development Goals (2023) Available at: https://www.undp.org/sustainable-development-goals?gclid=CjwKCAjw04yjBhApEiwAJcvNoQ1wagmkKECnNZqh286IJ23nL9RCgZQ36KovVitg6pOa9tZ7f_ZJGhoCVkEQAvD_BwE. Accessed 16 May 2023

Trivedi N et al (2019) Awareness of palliative care among a nationally representative sample of U.S. adults. J Palliat Med 22(12):1578–1582. https://doi.org/10.1089/jpm.2018.0656

Vogt J et al (2021) Symptom burden and palliative care needs of patients with incurable cancer at diagnosis and during the disease course. Oncologist 26(6):e1058–e1065. https://doi.org/10.1002/onco.13751

Wittenberg E, Reb A, Kanter E (2018) Communicating with patients and families around difficult topics in cancer care using the COMFORT communication curriculum. Semin Oncol Nurs 34(3):264–273. https://doi.org/10.1016/j.soncn.2018.06.007

Zhu Y, Engui S (2019) When patients say they know about palliative care, how much do they really understand? 58(3):460–464. https://doi.org/10.1016/j.jpainsymman.2019.05.008

Zimmermann C (2004) Denial of impending death: a discourse analysis of the palliative care literature. Soc Sci Med 59(8):1769–1780. https://doi.org/10.1016/j.socscimed.2004.02.012

Zimmermann C, Mathews J (2022) Palliative care is the umbrella, not the rain – a metaphor to guide conversations in advanced cancer. JAMA Oncol 8(5):681–682

Zimmermann C et al (2016) Perceptions of palliative care among patients with advanced cancer and their caregivers. CMAJ 188(10). https://doi.org/10.1503/cmaj.160206

Part IV
Concluding Remarks

Chapter 12
Conclusion

Marit Kvangarsnes, Bodil J. Landstad, Elise Kvalsund Bårdsgjerde, and Torstein Hole

Abstract The United Nations has warned that there is a lack of progress in reaching the Sustainable Development Goals (SDGs), affecting the world's poorest and most vulnerable people. These global challenges mean that the need for increasing levels of health literacy is more urgent than ever. Our responses to this are covered from a historical perspective in Parts I and II, alongside key aspects relevant to clinical practice and research. A comprehensive model for patient participation with a new perspective relevant to both research and practice is also presented. An overview of relevant qualitative research models is also described: this type of approach may provide a greater in-depth understanding of patients' experiences of various diseases. Transforming our world for sustainable development requires a systematic and a pedagogical approach to health literacy. To this end, we examine a pedagogical model for building health literacy alongside a strategy to improve supervision. Part III showcases studies to exemplify the importance of health literacy in different non-communicable diseases and from different perspectives. To conclude, we argue that the way forward for health literacy and strategies is to increase the emphasis on

M. Kvangarsnes (✉)
Department of Health Sciences in Ålesund, Norwegian University of Science and Technology (NTNU), Ålesund, Norway

Medical Department, Ålesund Hospital, Møre og Romsdal Hospital Trust, Ålesund, Norway
e-mail: marit.kvangarsnes@ntnu.no

B. J. Landstad
Department of Health Sciences, Mid Sweden University, Östersund, Sweden

Unit of Research, Education and Development, Östersund Hospital, Östersund, Sweden

E. K. Bårdsgjerde
Department of Health Sciences in Ålesund, Norwegian University of Science and Technology (NTNU), Ålesund, Norway

T. Hole
Medical Department, Ålesund Hospital, Møre og Romsdal Hospital Trust, Ålesund, Norway

Faculty of Medicine and Health Sciences, Norwegian University of Science and Technology (NTNU), Trondheim, Norway

T. Hole et al. (eds.), *Towards Sustainable Good Health and Well-being*,
https://doi.org/10.1007/978-3-031-61810-9_12

this area in current SDGs, and within future policies set for achieving these SDGs. These steps would serve to increase health literacy across the globe.

Keywords SDGs · Mortality · Non-communicable diseases · Patient participation · Digital healthcare · Innovative strategies · Health services

The climate crisis, wars, a weak global economy, and the effects of the COVID-19 pandemic have led to uncertainty and challenges globally. The United Nations (UN) has warned that there is a lack of progress in reaching the Sustainable Development Goals (SDGs) and that this affects the world's poorest and most vulnerable people (United Nations 2023). The need for health literacy is more urgent than ever to contend with such global challenges. This book contributes to a framework that can be used to strengthen health literacy and increase the possibility of achieving the associated SDGs.

SDGs are systematically measured and monitored for progress (WHO 2013b, 2024; United Nations 2015a; Our World in Data team 2023). The European Health Literacy Survey provides valuable data in improving health literacy worldwide. Data from this survey enables comparisons both within, and between, countries and has identified major inequities among populations (WHO 2013b, 2021). Throughout this book, we have considered it especially important to identify vulnerable groups in promoting equity for all people of all ages, aligned with the important principle of leaving no one behind (United Nations 2016, 2018).

Statistics have shown a strong decline in mortality from non-communicable diseases such as cancer, cardiovascular disease, diabetes, and chronic lung disease in Western countries. The decline has slowed down considerably during the last years, probably due to a lower number of smokers: policies/regulations have been introduced in many countries to support stopping smoking. Now the concern for the population is linked to other lifestyle factors, such as physical inactivity, unhealthy diet, and harmful use of alcohol (Ariansen and Larsen 2024). The UN's Sustainable Development Goal Good health and well-being (SDG 3) aims to reduce early death from non-communicable diseases by 33% in the period 2015–2030 (WHO 2013a; United Nations 2015b). This book has looked at challenges linked to health literacy for patients with non-communicable diseases. We found that there is a need for health professionals and health organisations alike to be aware of the importance of improving health literacy for patients, users, and their families. In-hospital health services are not accessible to all patients and end users: there is a need for systems to be adaptable to individual needs alongside digital healthcare services. This builds on previous findings that many patients and users will benefit from user-friendly electronic patient portals and training on how to use them (WHO 2013b).

Chapter 1 provided a historical backdrop to sustainability and the development of the sustainability goals. It demonstrated the interconnection between all 17 sustainability goals and highlighted the fact that reaching each of these 17 goals requires a multidisciplinary approach. The wedding cake model used in this opening chapter (Fig. 1.1) served to show that achieving good health and well-being

(SDG 3) is linked to the biosphere, society, and economic level. The top of the 'cake' shows that partnership and collaboration is key to achieving all the SDGs. This thread underpinned the thinking throughout the chapters. We have sought to show that the interaction between the individual and environment is crucial for the successful development of health literacy.

Improving health literacy requires patient participation and reduced inequalities among patients and health personnel. In western countries, there is comprehensive research on patient participation. Chapter 2 presented a model that added frame factors as a new perspective in research and practice in order to understand the complexity of patient participation and equality globally. We believe that there is great potential for this comprehensive model in studying patient participation in different cultures and healthcare systems.

It is important to develop knowledge about patients' experiences of illness, treatment, and health literacy so that health education can be adapted for various groups and patients' preferences. A qualitative research approach may therefore provide a greater in-depth understanding of patients' experiences of various diseases. Chapter 3 highlighted different qualitative designs and methods for exploring health literacy from various perspectives. Knowledge from the patient and end user perspective is certain to be transferable and particularly valuable when working towards the aim of achieving person-centred health education and health literate–friendly organisations.

Transforming our world for sustainable development requires a systematic and a pedagogical approach to health literacy. To this end, Chap. 4 presented a pedagogical model and framework for building health literacy for obtaining good health and well-being and sustainable health services at a personal and an organisational level. This pedagogical model employs an ecological approach which means that the engagement of individuals, social networks, organisations, communities, and the population continues to be essential in the quest to build health literacy.

We have also explored supervision, which is known to be important in improving health literacy among patients and health personnel. Chapter 5 therefore presented a supervision strategy which can be used to make individuals and organisations aware of the knowledge, experiences, and values underpinning their practice. The pedagogical model and the supervision strategy complement each other, and we sought to show how valuable they are when planning, implementing, and assessing health education individually and in groups. Both Chaps. 4 and 5 are important resources for use in medical, health, and social education. Health literacy is a new and important learning outcome across the curricula.

Enhancing health literacy through sustainable digital healthcare solutions requires a comprehensive strategy, in which patients, users, family caregivers, healthcare professionals, IT engineers, and technicians must participate and collaborate. The findings in Chap. 6 highlighted that it is essential that digital health services are user-friendly at both individual and system levels. Furthermore, it concludes that digital health services ought to also be intuitive and adapted to any age-related cognitive and physical challenges.

Throughout Part III in particular, we felt it important to highlight health literacy from the point of view of various stakeholders, like patients, family caregivers, and health professionals. Experiences from patients with non-communicable diseases, users with visual impairment, and health personnel can bestow us with invaluable knowledge on how to create a health literate–friendly environment. Chapters 7, 8, and 9 dealt with experiences of health literacy during both clinical pathways and life. We have endeavoured to show that health literacy and levels of health literacy are based on context and that educational needs vary in the clinical pathway and over a person's lifetime.

In Chap. 9, the sole informant is also a co-author. The experiences from this study showed that a user can contribute to different roles in research. The possibilities as well as the limitations with one of the researchers being both informant and co-author are discussed. The user's important role has strengthened the trustworthiness of the study and contributed to relevant suggestions for improving the learning environment for the visually impaired.

Chapter 10 dealt with how to improve health literacy among immigrant women, while Chap. 11 discussed health literacy in palliative care. The chapters discussed the importance of health literacy for quality in palliative care and how innovative strategies, used in other walks of life, could be applied to groups of immigrant women to increase their health literacy. Once again, these approaches are potentially highly transferable and adaptable for different health services and groups.

During our work on this book, we have gained a great deal of insight into the value of health literacy as a prerequisite for patient participation and as a way of empowering persons and communities to manage challenges. Health-literate people and organisations will render people better equipped to make better-informed decisions related to their health and well-being.

Finally, looking forward, we would question whether health literacy should actually be more explicitly and clearly stated in the 17 current sustainability goals. Extrapolating from the findings in these chapters, we believe that increasing levels of health literacy will affect the entire population's understanding and knowledge of a range of different areas. This could lend itself to, for example, an improved understanding about clean water and sanitation, nutrition, as well as the promotion of healthy environments. This may, in turn, lead to the achievement of SDG targets such as reducing infant and child mortality, preventing the spread of infectious diseases and the development of epidemics, and reducing mortality from non-communicable diseases as well as promoting mental health. We would therefore argue that health literacy and strategies to increase health literacy globally should be more clearly emphasised in the SDGs and in future policies which will be developed to achieve these SDGs.

References

Ariansen I, Larsen IK (2024) For tidlig død av ikke-smittsomme sykdommer [Premature mortality of non-communicable diseases]. Tidsskrift Nor Legeforen 2. https://doi.org/10.4045/tidsskr.23.0849

Our World in Data team (2023) SDG tracker: measuring progress towards the sustainable development goals. Available https://ourworldindata.org/sdgs. Accessed 21 Feb 2024

United Nations (2015a) Indicators and a monitoring framework for the sustainable development goals. Available https://sdgs.un.org/sites/default/files/publications/2013150612-FINAL-SDSN-Indicator-Report1.pdf. Accessed 21 Feb 2024

United Nations (2015b) Transforming our world: the 2030 Agenda for Sustainable development. Available https://sustainabledevelopment.un.org/content/documents/21252030%20Agenda%20for%20Sustainable%20Development%20web.pdf. Accessed 21 Feb 2024

United Nations (2016) Leaving no one behind: equality and non-discrimination at the heart of sustainable development. Available https://unsceb.org/sites/default/files/imported_files/CEB%20equality%20framework-A4-web-rev3.pdf. Accessed 21 Feb 2024

United Nations (2018) Leaving no one behind. Available https://sustainabledevelopment.un.org/content/documents/2754713_July_PM_2._Leaving_no_one_behind_Summary_from_UN_Committee_for_Development_Policy.pdf. Accessed 21 Feb 2024

United Nations (2023) The sustainable development goals report. Special edition. Available https://unstats.un.org/sdgs/report/2023/The-Sustainable-Development-Goals-Report-2023.pdf. Accessed 21 Feb 2024

WHO (2013a) Global action plan for the prevention and control of noncommunicable diseases 2013–2020. Available https://iris.who.int/bitstream/handle/10665/94384/9789241506236_eng.pdf?sequence=1. Accessed 21 Feb 2024

WHO (2013b) Health literacy The solid facts. Available https://apps.who.int/iris/bitstream/handle/10665/128703/e96854.pdf. Accessed 28 Aug 2023

WHO (2021) Short summary of the international report on the methodology, results, and recommendations of the European Health Literacy Population Survey 2019–2021 (HLS19) of M-POHL. Available https://m-pohl.net/sites/m-pohl.net/files/inline-files/HLS19%20Short%20Summary.pdf. Accessed 22 Feb 2024

WHO (2024) The global health observatory Explore a world of health data. Available https://www.who.int/data/gho/publications/world-health-statistics. Accessed 22 Feb 2024

Correction to: Empowering Agency: Enhancing Health Literacy Among Migrant Women Through Health Parties: A Case Study

Marianne Hedlund, Yan Zhao, and Trude Karine Olaug Gjernes

Correction to:
Chapter 10 in: T. Hole et al. (eds.),
***Towards Sustainable Good Health and Well-being*,**
https://doi.org/10.1007/978-3-031-61810-9_10

The first name of Yan Zhao was unfortunately published with an error. The initially published version has now been corrected.

The updated version of this chapter can be found at
https://doi.org/10.1007/978-3-031-61810-9_10

T. Hole et al. (eds.), *Towards Sustainable Good Health and Well-being*,
https://doi.org/10.1007/978-3-031-61810-9_13

